Pediatric Assessment

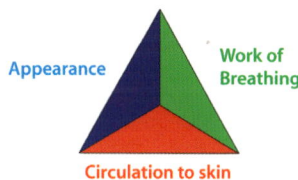

The Pediatric Assessment Triangle

Used with permission of the American Academy of Pediatrics, *Pediatric Education for Prehospital Professionals*, Copyright American Academy of Pediatrics, 2000.

Appearance

Mental status

Muscle tone

Body position

Breathing

Visible movement

Work of breathing (normal/increased)

Circulation

Color

W0113637

■ Pediatric Emergencies—General Assessment

Airway: Look for obstruction, drooling, trauma, edema.

Breathing: Retractions? Respiratory rate? Good air movement?

Circulation: Heart rate? Capillary refill?

Bradycardia means hypoxia. Ventilate!

Mental Status: Is Child Acting Normally?

Hx—Present illness/onset, intake, GI habits. Perform examination: Fever? Skin color? Other findings?

Children in shock need aggressive treatment.

- Ventilate. Reassess the airway, especially during transport.
- Check CBG, consider naloxone.
- IV fluid challenge (20 mL/kg—repeat if necessary.) Do not wait for BP to drop—hypotension is a late sign.
- Rapid transport to a pediatric intensive care facility.

Cautions—Not every seizure with fever is a febrile seizure.

- Consider meningitis, especially in children < 2 yo (check for a rash that does not blanch).
- Early signs of sepsis are subtle: grunting respirations, temperature instability, hypoglycemia, poor feeding, etc.
- Consider toxins.

Croup

Hx—Cold or flu that develops into a **"barking cough"** at night. Relatively slow onset. Low fever.

Treatment— Fluids, cool mist, nebulized racemic epinephrine. Transport to ED.

Cautions—Do not examine the upper airway.

Epiglottitis

Hx—Cold or flu that develops into a high fever at night. **Drooling, difficulty swallowing**, relatively rapid onset. Inspiratory stridor may be present in severe cases.

Treatment—O₂, place patient in position of comfort. If airway becomes completely obstructed, ventilate with BVM, prepare for ET intubation.

Cautions—Do not examine the upper airway. This may cause total airway obstruction. Some patients with epiglottitis deteriorate rapidly, requiring ventilation, intubation, or cricothyrotomy.

Croup Versus Epiglottitis

	Croup	Epiglottitis
Age	< 3 yo	2–6 yo
Sex	♂ / ♀	Both ♂ and ♀
Onset	Gradual (at night)	Relatively rapid
Infection	Viral	Bacterial (Hib)
Fever	Low grade	High fever
Breathing	Retractions	Tripod: sitting, leaning forward
Sounds	"Barking cough"	Inspiratory stridor
Voice	Hoarseness	Muffled voice
Other S/Sx		Drooling, painful swallowing
Treatment	Fluids, cool mist, nebulized Rx, may need steroids or racemic epinephrine in the hospital	O₂, position of comfort, may need intubation or cricothyrotomy in the hospital **Do not examine airway**

Because children are now being routinely immunized for Hib, epiglottitis is actually more common in adults than children.

RSV (Respiratory Syncytial Virus)

Hx—Affects all ages; most common cause of lower respiratory tract infection (LRTI) in children < 1 yo. More common during flu season. Infection does not incur immunity. Infants/children usually present with bronchiolitis, LRTI, or pneumonia. 20% of infants develop RSV wheezing in 1st yr; may lead to apnea. Children/adults may have upper or lower respiratory s/s.

Treatment—Supportive care, bronchodilators, fluids, transport to ED. Apnea or severe cases may need respiratory support.

Normal Pediatric Vital Signs

Age	Resp.	Pulse	SBP*	Weight	Weight
Preterm	40–60	140	50–60	3 lbs	1.5 kg
Term NB	40–60	125	70	7 lbs	3.5 kg
6 months	24–36	120	90	15 lbs	7 kg
1 year old	22–30	120	95	22 lbs	10 kg
3 years old	20–26	110	100	33 lbs	15 kg
6 years old	20–24	100	100	44 lbs	20 kg
8 years old	18–22	90	105	55 lbs	25 kg
10 years old	18–22	90	110	66 lbs	30 kg
12 years old	16–22	85	115	88 lbs	40 kg
14 years old	14–20	80	115	99 lbs	45 kg

* SBP = systolic blood pressure

■ Formulas for Pediatric Vital Signs

Newborn (first 72 hours): Normal mean arterial pressure (MAP) = gestational age (GA) in weeks (i.e., 30-week infant; normal MAP 30 mmHg). MAP < 18 or MAP > (GA - 5 mmHg) suggests hypoperfusion (correlate with clinical s/s such as cap refill).

Infants < 1 yo: Minimum SBP of 60 mmHg

Infants/Children > 1 yo: Minimum SBP = 70 mmHg + (2 × age in years)

Pediatric Trauma Score				
	+ 2	+ 1	−1	Score
Patient size	>20 kg	10–20 kg	<10 kg	
Airway	Normal	Maintainable without invasive procedures	Not maintainable, NEEDS invasive procedures	
CNS	Awake	Obtunded	Comatose	
Systolic BP (mm Hg) (or pulse)	>90 (radial)	50–90 (femoral)	<50 (no pulse)	
Open wounds	None	Minor	Major or penetrating	
Skeletal	None	Closed Fx	Open/multiple fracture	
			Total =	
9–12 = Minor trauma (9% mortality)				
6–8 = Potentially life threatening				
0–5 = Life threatening				
≤ 0 = Usually fatal (100% mortality)				

Glasgow Coma Scale

NOTE: A score of 3 is considered a coma; ≤8 requires intubation and airway management.

INFANT		Eye Opening		CHILD/ADULT
	4	Spontaneously	Spontaneously	4
	3	To speech	To command	3
	2	To pain	To pain	2
_____	1	No response	No response	1 _____
		Best Verbal Response		
	5	Coos, babbles	Oriented	5
	4	Irritable cries	Confused	4
	3	Cries to pain	Inappropriate words	3
	2	Moans, grunts	Incomprehensible	2
_____	1	No response	No response	1 _____
		Best Motor Response		
	6	Spontaneous	Obeys commands	6
	5	Localizes pain	Localizes pain	5
	4	Withdraws from pain	Withdraws from pain	4
	3	Flexion (decorticate)	Flexion (decorticate)	3
	2	Extension (decerebrate)	Extension (decerebrate)	2
_____	1	No response	No response	1 _____
_____		= Total	(GCS score ≤8? → Intubate!)	Total = _____

(Continues)

Interpretation of GCS:	
15:	Normal
13–14:	Minor injury to head
9–12:	Moderate injury to head
3–8:	Severe injury to head
4–7:	Coma may be present
3:	Deep coma or brain death

◼ Intraosseous Infusion

NOTE: Most medications, blood products, or solutions that can be given IV can be given IO.

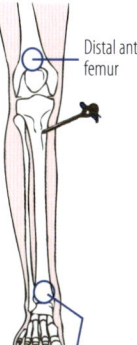

Distal anterior femur

1. **Locate anterior medial (flat) surface of tibia, 2 cm below tibial tuberosity, below growth plate (other sites: distal anterior femur, medial malleolus, iliac crest).**
2. **Prep area with antiseptic solution.**
3. Advance IO needle at 90° angle through skin, fascia, and bone with constant pressure and twisting motion. Direct needle slightly away from epiphyseal plate.
4. **A popping sensation will occur** (and a lack of resistance) **when you have reached the marrow space.**
5. **Attempt to aspirate marrow** (you may or may not get marrow).

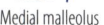

Medial malleolus

6. **Infuse fluids and check for infiltration.** Discontinue if site becomes infiltrated with fluid or medications, apply manual pressure to site followed by a pressure dressing.
7. Secure IO needle, tape in place, and attach to IV pump.

7

Airway Management

RESUSCITATE BEFORE YOU INTUBATE. Normalize vital signs.

◼ Mnemonics

Patient Assessment

A—Airway
B—Breathing
C—Circulation
D—Disability
E—Expose

Rapid Triage

A—Alert
V—Responds to Verbal
P—Responds to Pain
U—Unresponsive

Altered Mental Status

A—Alcohol/Drugs
E—Endocrine
I—Insulin/Infection
O—Overdose
U—Uremla

T—Trauma
I—Infection
P—Psychiatric
S—Shock

Pain Questions

O—Onset
P—Provoke/Palliative
Q—Quality/Character
R—Region or Radiation
S—Signs/Symptoms/
   Severity
T—Time of Onset/
   Duration/Intensity

History-Taking

S—Signs and Symptoms
A—Allergies
M—Medications
P—Pertinent Past History
L—Last Meal
E—Events

Newborn Assessment

A—Appearance
P—Pulse
G—Grimace
A—Activity
R—Respirations

■ CPAP : Continuous Positive Airway Pressure

- ■ Treats shortness of breath 2° to increase work of breathing (WOB)
- ■ CPAP is non-invasive ventilation (NIV)
- ■ Disposable units are most common in EMS

Indications:
- ■ Any patient in respiratory distress with increased WOB
- ■ CPAP is okay for kids

Contraindications:
- ■ Apnea (need BVM assist)
- ■ Unable to protect airway/vomiting/excessive secretions
- ■ Inability to obtain mask seal

Mask Placement:

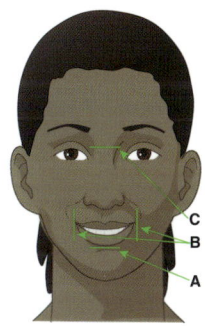

The mask should cover:
a. Below the lower lip with the mouth open
b. Corners of the mouth
c. Just below the junction of the nasal cartilage and bone

9

- Mask should not be too tight **(there will be a leak)**
- Masks have anti-asphyxia valves so patient can still breath during gas loss

"Selling CPAP"

1. Patients with shortness of breath (SOB) are anxious; use a calm, reassuring approach
2. Hand the mask to the patient so they can place it on their face
3. Usual starting pressure is 8-10 CWP; titrate up to effect once in place
4. Apply headgear once mask is in place and patient is comfortable
5. Provide continued reassurance

Reassessment Pearls:

- Subjective: BORG scale (rate SOB from 0-10)
- Objective:
  - ❑ $\downarrow$ RR
  - ❑ $\uparrow$ SpO_2
  - ❑ $\downarrow$ $EtCO_2$*
  - ❑ $\downarrow$ WOB

*$EtCO_2$ best obtained using nasal cannula w/ oral pillow, placed under mask

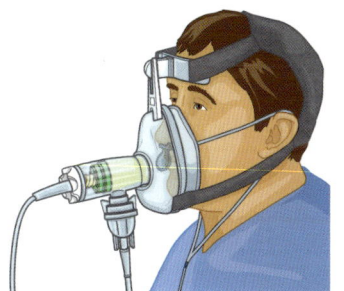

■ Reasonable trial of CPAP is 20 min. If there is no improvement, consider BVM assist.

■ i-gel Supraglottic Airway

Contraindications—Intact gag reflex, upper airway obstruction, trismus, caustic ingestions.
1. **Preoxygenate with 100% O_2.**
2. **Choose proper size (see chart).**

i-gel Sizing Chart			
Package Color	Patient Size	Size	Weight
Orange	Large adult	5	90+ kg
Green	Medium adult	4	50–90 kg
Yellow	Small adult	3	30–60 kg
White	Large pediatric	2.5	25–35 kg
Grey	Small pediatric	2	10–25 kg
Blue	Infant	1.5	5 12 kg
Pink	Neonate	1	2–5 kg

Airway

3. **Place lubricant into middle of smooth surface of cradle, and lubricate back, sides, and front of cuff with a thin layer.**
4. **Place patient in sniffing position.**
5. **Grasp i-gel by bite block, insert until definitive resistance is felt.**
6. **Secure in place, ventilate with BVM.**
7. **Verify proper placement:**
   - Check chest expansion and lung sounds
   - Apply waveform capnography, oximetry
   - Reassess periodically

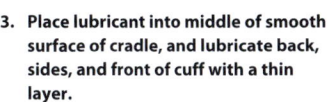

■ King LTS-D Airway

Contraindications—Does not protect against aspiration.

1. **C-spine immobilization**, as needed.
   Preoxygenate with 100% O_2. Apply water-based lubricant to distal tip and posterior aspect of tube.
2. **Deflate cuff. Open mouth, apply chin lift, insert tip** into side of mouth.

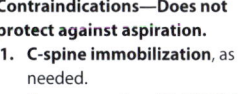

3. **Advance tip** behind tongue while rotating tube to midline.

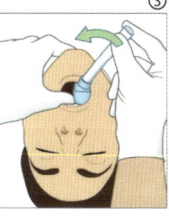

4. **Advance tube** until base of connector is aligned with teeth or gums.

5. **Inflate cuff** with air (see chart; use minimum volume necessary).

Patient Size	LTS-D Size	Cuff Volume (mL)
NB < 5 kg	0	10
Infant 5 – 12 kg	1	20
12–25 kg	2	35
25–35 kg	2.5	40–45
4–5 ft	3	50–60
5–6 ft	4	70–80
>6 ft	5	80–90

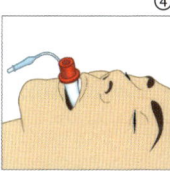

6. **Attach BVM.** While ventilating, gently adjust tube until ventilation becomes easy (i.e., good chest rise and fall).

7. **Adjust cuff inflation**, if necessary, to obtain a good seal (max 60 cm H_2O).

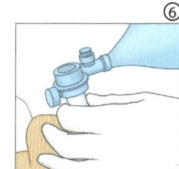

8. **Verify proper placement:**
   - Check chest expansion and lung sounds.
   - Apply CO_2 detector; oximeter.
   - Secure with tape or tube holder.
   - Reassess airway periodically.

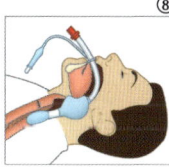

Airway

Bag-Valve Mask Technique

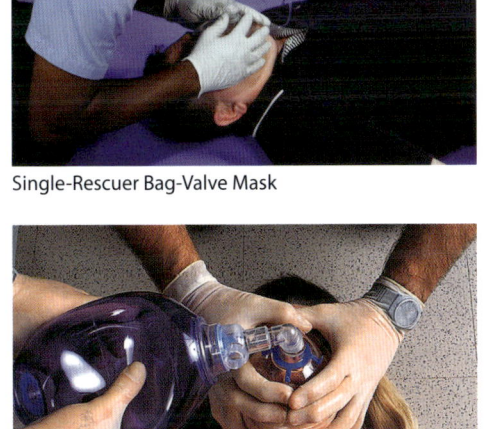

Single-Rescuer Bag-Valve Mask

Dual-Rescuer Bag-Valve Mask

Interpreting Capnography Waveforms

End-Tidal CO_2 Monitoring (Capnography)

Applications	Description	Waveform
Normal capnographic waveform	Four phases, plots CO_2 concentration over time AB = respiratory baseline BC = expiratory upstroke CD = expiratory plateau DE = inhalation of CO_2-free gas	
WARNING: Detect esophageal placement of ET tube during intubation!	A flat line occurs; no CO_2 is detected. Remove tube and ventilate with BVM or other advanced airway.	————————
Corresponds with ET tube placement in trachea	When tracheal placement occurs, exhaled CO_2 is shown on capnogram (35–45 mm Hg)	
Identify patient's attempt to breathe while paralyzed	Movement of patient's diaphragm results in a dip in the capnogram waveform	
WARNING: Indicates patient's disconnection from mechanical ventilator!	Waveform immediately disappears and goes flat	————————
Predictor of patient outcome	The higher the CO_2, the higher the cardiac output, and the more effective the resuscitation efforts	

Resuscitation

■ Cardiac Arrest Rhythms

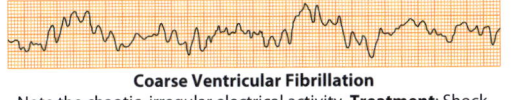

Coarse Ventricular Fibrillation
Note the chaotic, irregular electrical activity. **Treatment**: Shock.

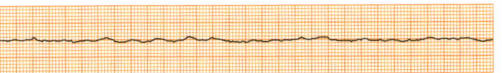

Fine Ventricular Fibrillation
Note the low-amplitude, irregular electrical activity. **Treatment**: Shock.

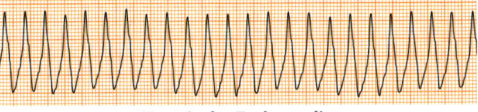

Ventricular Tachycardia
Note the rapid, wide complexes. **Treatment**: Shock if no pulse.

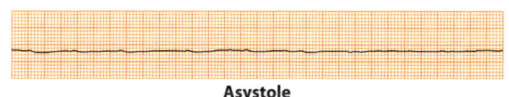

Asystole
Note the absence of electrical activity. **Treatment**: Perform CPR.

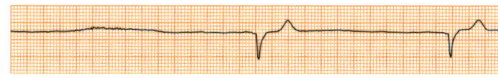

Pulseless Electrical Activity (PEA)
Any organized ECG rhythm with no pulse. **Treatment**: Perform CPR.

Other Common ECG Rhythms

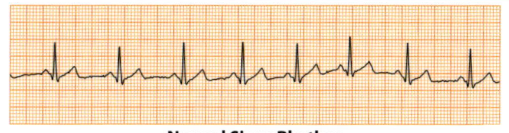

Normal Sinus Rhythm
Note the regular PQRST cycles.

Go to next page

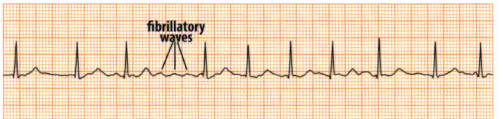

Atrial Fibrillation

Note the irregular rate and atrial fibrillatory waves.

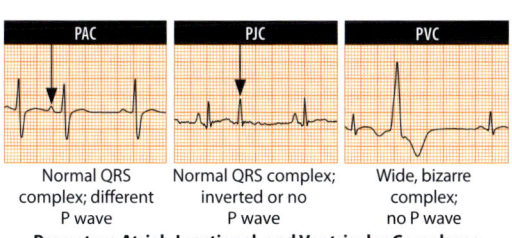

PAC	PJC	PVC
Normal QRS complex; different P wave	Normal QRS complex; inverted or no P wave	Wide, bizarre complex; no P wave

Premature Atrial, Junctional, and Ventricular Complexes

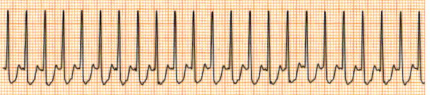

Supraventricular Tachycardia (SVT)

Note the rapid, narrow QRS complexes.

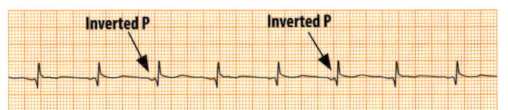

Junctional Rhythm
Normal QRS complexes; inverted or no P waves

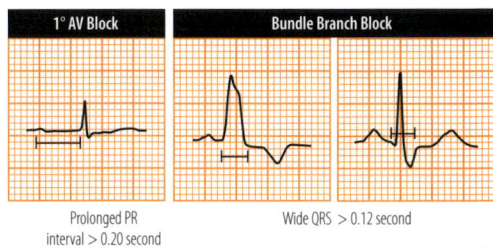

Prolonged PR
interval > 0.20 second

Wide QRS > 0.12 second

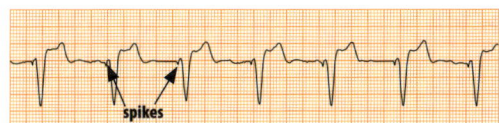

Electronic Ventricular Pacemaker
Note the pacer spikes before each QRS.

Basic ECG Interpretation

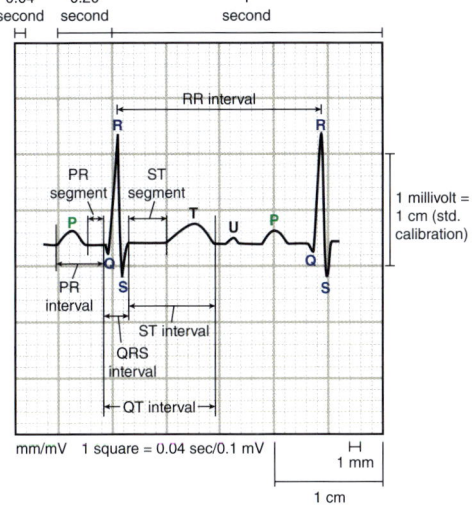

ECG Waves:
P Wave: Atrial depolarization
QRS Complex: Ventricular depolarization
T/U Waves: Ventricular repolarization

Normal duration of ECG segments:
PR interval: 0.12 – 0.2 secs (3-5 mm)
QRS: <0.12 secs (3 mm)
QTc: 0.38 – 0.42 secs (9-10 mm)

3-Lead and MCL₁ Electrode Placement

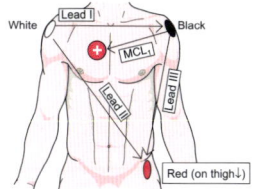
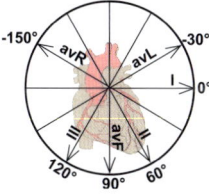

Chest Pain

Present Hx—Syncope, dizziness, weakness, diaphoresis, fever, pallor, dyspnea?

Past Hx—Chest trauma, cardiac or respiratory problems, diabetes, high blood pressure, heart failure, lung sounds, JVD, peripheral or pulmonary edema, general appearance?

Treatment: Position of comfort, reassure patient, vitals, O_2, ECG, IV. Consider nitroglycerin for cardiac chest pain: 0.4 mg SL every 5 minutes (maximum: 3 doses). Consider aspirin for AMI.

IMPORTANT: Notify ED if your cardiac patient is a possible fibrinolytic candidate, and transport ASAP.

Cautions—Treat dysrhythmias according to ACLS.

Resuscitation

4-lead: Smoke over Fire, Cloud over Grass

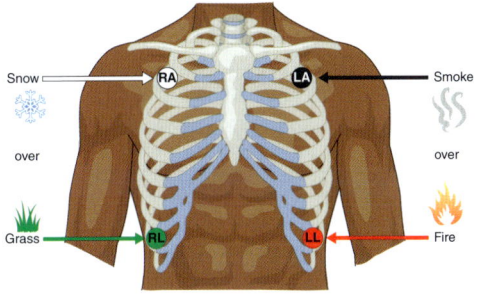

Snow → RA LA ← Smoke

over   over

Grass → RL LL ← Fire

Consider:

- **Acute MI:** Severe, crushing chest pain, or substernal "pressure," radiating to the left arm or jaw. N/V, SOB, diaphoresis, pallor, dysrhythmias, HTN or hypotension

- **Aortic Dissection:** Sudden onset "tearing" chest or back pain, tachycardia, HTN or hypotension, diaphoresis, possible unequal pulses or unequal BP in extremities

- **Cholelithiasis:** Acute onset RUQ pain and tenderness (may be referred to right shoulder/scapula)—may be related to high-fat meal; N/V, anorexia, fever.

Go to next page

- **Hiatal Hernia:** Positional epigastric pain
- **Musculoskeletal:** Pain on palpation, respiration. Obvious signs of trauma
- **Pleurisy:** Pain on inspiration, fever, pleural friction rub
- **Pneumonia:** Fever, shaking, chills, pleuritic chest pain, crackles, productive cough, tachycardia, diaphoresis
- **Pulmonary Embolus:** Sudden onset SOB, cough, chest pain that is sharp and pleuritic, tachycardia, rapid respirations, O_2 sat < 94%, apprehension, diaphoresis, hemoptysis, crackles
- **Ulcer/GERD:** "Burning" epigastric pain, N/V, possible hematemesis, hypotension, decreased bowel sounds

Resuscitation

ACLS Algorithms

NOTE: Not all patients require the treatment indicated by these algorithms. These algorithms assume that you have assessed the patient, started CPR where indicated, and performed reassessment after each treatment. These algorithms also do not exclude other appropriate interventions that may be warranted by the patient's condition.

Treat the patient, not the ECG.

Positions for 6-Person High-Performance Teams*

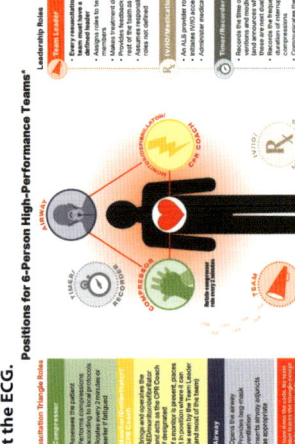

*This is a suggested team formation. Roles may be adapted to local protocol.

© 2020 American Heart Association

■ Cardiac Arrest

Shout for help, begin CPR (30:2, push hard and fast
at 100–120/min., minimize interruptions), **give O₂, attach ECG.**
YES ← Shockable Rhythm? → **NO**

VF or VT	Asystole/PEA

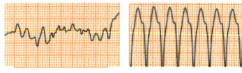

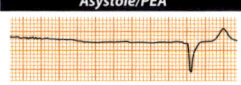

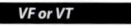 **Defibrillate 120 J–200 J** **Biphasic** (or 360 J monophasic, or AED)	**Continue CPR immediately.** X 2 minutes. Start IV/IO. **ASAP Epinephrine**, 1 mg IV/IO, repeat every 3–5 minutes, consider advanced airway **Ventilate** 8–10 breaths/minute with continuous compressions
↓	↓
Continue CPR immediately × 2 minutes. Start IV/IO	Asystole/PEA? **Continue CPR** × 2 minutes Consider and treat reversible causes*
↓	↓
Consideration of Supraglottic airway after first round of CPR and defibrillation	If ROSC (pulse, BP, PETCO₂ ≥40 mm Hg), see *ROSC algorithm*, next page.
↓	

VF/VT?
↓
〽 **Defibrillate** **Continue CPR** × 2 minutes Epinephrine, 1 mg IV/IO, repeat every 3–5 minutes. **Ventilate** 8–10 breaths/minute with continuous compressions
↓

VF/VT?
〽 **Defibrillate** **Continue CPR** × 2 minutes Consider and treat reversible causes*
↓
If ROSC (pulse, BP, PETCO₂ ≥40 mm Hg), see *ROSC algorithm*, next page

*Reversible Causes

- Hypoxia
- Hypovolemia
- Acidosis
- Hyper-/hypokalemia
- Hypothermia
- Coronary thrombosis
- Pulmonary thrombosis
- Cardiac tamponade
- Tension pneumothorax
- Toxins

25

Resuscitation

■ Return of Spontaneous Circulation: Post-Cardiac Arrest Care

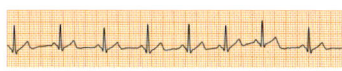

Optimize ventilation/oxygenation
Early placement of advanced airway; start ventilation at 10 breaths/min.

Use minimum amount of FiO_2 to keep SaO_2 ≥ 92–98%

↓

Keep blood pressure > 90 mm Hg (or MAP > 65 mm Hg)

IV fluid bolus: 1–2 L NS or RL
(May use cold [4°C] IV fluid if induced hypothermia)

Consider and treat reversible causes*

Monitor ECG

Follows commands?

↓

Transport to PCI-capable center

*Reversible Causes

- Hypoxia
- Acidosis
- Hypovolemia
- Toxins
- Coronary thrombosis

- Cardiac tamponade
- Hyper-/hypokalemia
- Hypothermia
- Pulmonary thrombosis
- Tension pneumothorax

Field Determination of Death

EMS Clinical Exam for Death:
- Time of assessment (this is the time of death)
- No response to verbal or tactile stimulation
- No pupillary light reflex (pupils fixed and dilated)
- Absence of breath sounds
- Absence of heart sounds
- AED or ECG = no signs of life

EMS Death Documentation:
- Describe your exam
- Location/position where found
- Physical condition of body
- Significant medical Hx or trauma
- Conditions precluding resuscitation
- Any medical control contact
- Person body left in custody of

Tips:
- Following field termination of resuscitation, observe patient for at least 10 minutes for autoresuscitation (return of vital signs).
- Isolated fatal injuries may be candidates for organ donation.
- Some patients underwater for less than 2 hours have survived (never > 2 hours).
- Beware of hypothermia, cannot declare death until core temp > 90°F.
- ALS providers should record a rhythm strip; leave electrodes on the body and a copy of the strip with the body.

Resuscitation

Asthma Cardiac Arrest

Use standard ACLS guidelines
↓

To reduce hyperinflation, hypotension, and risk of tension pneumothorax, consider:

- **Ventilation with a slower respiratory rate**
- **Smaller tidal volume (6–8 mL/kg)**
- **Shorter inspiratory time (<= 0.5 seconds)**
- **Longer expiratory time (I/E 1:4 or 1:5)**

↓

Continue use of **inhaled β_2-agonist (albuterol)** via ET tube
Evaluate for tension pneumothorax

↓

Consult with expert
Consider brief disconnect from BVM and press on chest wall during exhalation to relieve air trapping

↓

If the patient suddenly deteriorates:

↓

DOPE

- Displacement of ET tube
- Obstruction of tube
- Pneumothorax
- Equipment failure
- Evaluate for Auto-PEEP

Drowning Cardiac Arrest

- **Begin rescue breathing ASAP.**
- Start CPR with A-B-C (airway and breathing first).
- Anticipate vomiting (have suction ready).
- Attach AED (dry chest off with towel).
- **Check for hypothermia.**
- **Use standard BLS and ACLS.**

Electrocution Cardiac Arrest

Respiratory arrest is common.

- **Is the scene safe?**
- **Triage patients and treat those with respiratory arrest or cardiac arrest first.**
- Start CPR.
- Stabilize the cervical spine.
- Attach AED.
- **Remove smoldering clothing.**
- Check for trauma.
- **Use large-bore IV catheter for rapid fluid administration.**
- Consider advanced airway for airway burns.
- **Use standard BLS and ACLS.**

Trauma Cardiac Arrest

- Direct pressure for hemorrhage.
- Jaw thrust to open airway.
- **Stabilize cervical spine.**
- Consider and treat reversible causes*.
- **Perform standard CPR and defibrillation.**
- **Use advanced airway if BVM inadequate** (consider cricothyrotomy if ventilation impossible).
- **Administer IV fluids** for hypovolemia.

*Reversible Causes

Hypoxia	Coronary thrombosis	Pulmonary thrombosis
Acidosis	Cardiac tamponade	Tension pneumothorax
Hypovolemia	Hyper-/hypokalemia	
Toxins	Hypothermia	

"Commotio cordis": a blow to the anterior chest causing VF

- **Prompt CPR and defibrillation**
- **Use standard BLS and ACLS.**

Hypothermia

- **Remove wet clothing and stop heat loss** (cover with blankets and insulating equipment).
- **Keep patient horizontal.**
- **Move patient gently, if possible;** do not jostle.
- **Monitor core temperature and cardiac rhythm.**
- Treat underlying causes (drug overdose, alcohol, trauma, etc.) simultaneously with resuscitation.
- **Check responsiveness, breathing, and pulse.**

If Pulse and Breathing	No Pulse/Apneic
34°C–36°C / 93°F–97°F (MILD rewarming) **Passive rewarming**	**Start CPR, ventilate** **Defibrillate VF/VT** **Resume CPR immediately** (Consider further defibrillation attempts for VF/VT) *See Cardiac Arrest Algorithm* **Intubate, ventilate with warm, humid oxygen (42°C–46°C)** **Start IV/IO fluids, administer warm normal saline (43°C)** (Consider vasopressor: epinephrine 1 mg IV/IO every 3–5 minutes)
30°C–34°C / 86°F–93°F (MODERATE hypothermia) **Active external rewarming** **Forced-air rewarming**	
< 30°C / < 86°F (SEVERE hypothermia) **Core rewarming**	

Adjunctive Rewarming

- Warm IV fluids (43°C)
- Warm, humid O_2 (42°C–46°C)

↓

Continue CPR, transport to ED, start core rewarming when feasible. Continue resuscitation until patient is rewarmed.

↓

After ROSC, rewarm patient to 32°C–34°C (90°F–93°F) or to normal body temperature.

Acute Coronary Syndromes

1. **Signs and symptoms suggestive of ischemia or infarction**

2. **EMS assessment**
   - ABCs, prepare for CPR; have defibrillator ready
   - Give oxygen, aspirin, NTG, start IV fluids
   - **Oxygen** if saturation <90%, start oxygen and titrate
   - **Aspirin,** 162–325 mg chewable
   - **Nitroglycerin,** 0.3–0.4 mg SL tablet, repeat q 5 mins × 3 doses or aerosol 1–2 sprays @ 5 min intervals, max: 3 sprays in 15 min.
   - Obtain 12-lead ECG; *if ST elevation*, notify hospital and transmit (STEMI alert).
   - Note time of onset and first medical contact.

CPR: Adult, Child, or Infant

1. **Unresponsive?** (Not breathing, or only gasping?)
2. **Call for assistance**—have someone get defibrillator/AED.
3. **Check pulse/breathing within 10 seconds** (If pulse is present, give 1 breath every 5–6 seconds; check pulse every 2 minutes).
4. **If opioid overdose suspected**, administer naloxone **0.04–0.4 mg IM or IV**, repeat every 2–3 min PRN; intranasal 2 mg, repeat every 3–5 min PRN.

IF NO PULSE:
5. **Position patient supine** on hard, flat surface.
6. **Begin chest compressions**, 30:2, push hard and fast (100–120/minute), allow full chest recoil—minimize interruptions.
7. **Open airway:** head-tilt/chin-lift, ventilate × 2 (avoid excessive ventilations).
8. **Attach AED**. (See next page.)

SHOCKABLE RHYTHM?

Yes

9. **Shock × 1**.
10. **Resume CPR immediately** for 2 minutes.
11. **Check rhythm**.

IF SHOCKABLE:
12. **Shock × 1**; resume CPR.

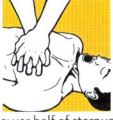

Lower half of sternum

No

9. **Resume CPR immediately** for 2 minutes.
10. **Epi ASAP/other ALS interventions**.
11. **Check rhythm** every 2 minutes.

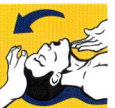

Head-tilt/chin-lift

CPR*	Ratio	Rate	Depth	Check Pulse
Adult: 1 Person	30:2	100–120	2–2.4 in.	Carotid
Adult: 2 Person	30:2	100–120	2–2.4 in.	Carotid
Child: 1 Person	30:2	100–120	2 in.	Carotid, femoral
Child: 2 Person	15:2	100–120	2 in.	Carotid, femoral
Infant: 1 Person	30:2	100–120	1/3 cx OR 1.5 in.	Brachial, femoral
Infant: 2 Person	15:2	100–120	1/3 cx OR 1.5 in.	Brachial, femoral
Newborn: 2 Person	3:1	100–120	1/3 cx OR 1.5 in.	Brachial, femoral

*With advanced airway: ventilate adults 10 breaths/min; infants/children 20–30 breaths/min.

■ Choking

For Responsive Choking Adult or Child >1 Year

1. If patient cannot talk or has stridor or cyanosis
2. **Perform Heimlich maneuver** (use chest thrusts if patient is pregnant or has obesity), repeat until successful or patient is unconscious
   If patient loses consciousness: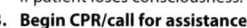
3. **Begin CPR/call for assistance**
4. Perform chest compressions (30:2)
5. Open airway—head-tilt/chin-lift (look and remove object, if visible)
6. Ventilate with 2 breaths. If unable . . .
7. Reposition head; attempt to ventilate. If unable . . .
8. Perform chest compressions (30:2)
9. Repeat: inspect mouth → remove object → ventilate → chest compressions **until successful**
10. Consider laryngoscopy and removal of object by forceps, ET intubation, transtracheal ventilation, cricothyrotomy
11. **If patient resumes breathing, place in the recovery position**

Resuscitation

For Unresponsive Choking Adult or Child

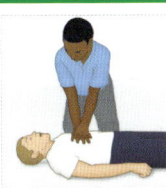

1. Determine unresponsiveness
2. Call for assistance
3. Position patient supine **on hard, flat surface**
4. Perform chest compressions (30:2)
5. Open airway—head-tilt/chin-lift (look and remove object if visible)
6. Attempt to ventilate. If unable . . .
7. Reposition head and chin; attempt to ventilate. If unable . . .
8. Perform chest compressions (30:2)
9. Repeat: inspect mouth → remove object → ventilate → chest compressions **until successful**
10. Consider laryngoscopy and removal of object by forceps, ET intubation, transtracheal ventilation, cricothyrotomy
11. **If patient resumes breathing, place in the recovery position**

For Choking Infant

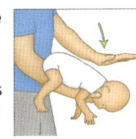

1. Confirm obstruction: **if infant cannot make sounds, breathe, cry, or is cyanotic**
2. Invert infant on arm: **support head by cupping face in hand;** perform 5 back slaps and 5 chest thrusts **until object is expelled**
3. Repeat until successful
4. If patient becomes unconscious, start CPR
5. Perform chest compressions (30:2)

6. Open airway, and ventilate with two breaths.
   If unable . . .
7. Reposition head and chin; attempt to ventilate again
8. Perform chest compressions (30:2)
9. Consider laryngoscopy and removal of object by forceps, ET intubation, transtracheal ventilation, cricothyrotomy
10. **If patient resumes breathing, place in the recovery position**

■ Childbirth

Hx—Timing of contractions? Intensity? Does mother have urge to push or to move bowels? Has amniotic sac ruptured? Medications—any medical problems? Vital signs, **check for:**

■ **Vaginal bleeding** or amniotic fluid; note color of fluid
■ **Crowning** (means imminent delivery)
■ **Abnormal presentation:** Foot, arm, breech, cord, shoulder
■ **Transport immediately** if patient has had previous C-section, known multiple births, any abnormal presentation, excessive bleeding, or if pregnancy is not full-term and child will be premature

Normal: Control delivery using gloved hand to guide head, suction mouth and nose, deliver, keep infant level with perineum, clamp and cut cord 8"–10" from infant, **warm and dry infant**, stimulate infant by drying with towel, **make sure respirations are adequate. Normal VS: pulse > 120 beats/minute; respiratory rate > 40 breaths/minute; BP 70 mm Hg; weight 3.5 kg.**

Give infant to mother to nurse at breast. Get Apgar scores at 1 and 5 minutes after birth.

If excessive postpartum bleeding, treat for shock, massage uterus to aid contraction, have mother nurse infant, *start large-bore IV catheter and consider oxytocin IV infusion or IM administration*, transport without waiting for placenta to deliver. Bring it with you to the hospital. Obtain mother's vital signs.

Most births are normal—reassure the mother.

Apgar Score					
	0 points	1 point	2 points	1 min	5 min
Color	Blue, pale	Body: pink Extremities: blue	Fully pink		
Heart rate	Absent	< 100	> 100		
Irritability	No response	Some	Vigorous		
Muscle tone	Flaccid	Some flexion of extremities	Active motion		
Respiratory effort	Absent	Slow, irregular	Strong cry		
			TOTAL =		

Infants with scores of 7–10 usually only need supportive care. **A score of 4–6 indicates moderate depression. Infants with scores of ≤ 3 require aggressive resuscitation.**

Breech: Call OLMC. If head will not deliver, consider applying gentle pressure on mother's abdomen. If unsuccessful, insert two gloved fingers in vagina between baby's face and vaginal wall to create airway. **Rapid transport.**

Cord Presents: Call OLMC. Place mother in Trendelenburg and knee-chest position, hold pressure on infant's head to relieve pressure on cord, check pulses in cord, keep cord moist with saline dressing, administer O_2, **begin rapid transport,** *start IV catheter en route.*

Foot/Leg Presentation: Call OLMC. Support presenting part, place mother in Trendelenburg and knee-chest position, administer O_2, **begin rapid transport, *start IV catheter en route.***

Cord Around Neck: Unwrap cord from neck and deliver normally, keep face clear, suction mouth and nose.

Infant Not Breathing: Stimulate with dry towel, rub back, flick soles of feet with finger. **Suction mouth and nose. Ventilate with BVM and 100% O_2** (this will revive most infants). **Begin chest compressions if HR < 60 bpm.** Ventilate with 100% O_2. If infant does not respond, contact OLMC and reassess quality of ventilation efforts, lung sounds (pneumothorax? obstruction?), check O_2 tube is connected. *Ventilate. Consider IV fluids, 10 mL/kg; glucose, 2 mL/kg D25%W; epinephrine, 0.01 mg/kg IV/IO.* **Rapid transport.** Failure to respond usually indicates hypoxia.

Medical Emergencies

■ Pain Assessment

10-Point Pain Scale		
Appearance	Pain Level	Score
	No Pain	0
	Mild Pain	1-3
	Moderate Pain	4-6
	Severe Pain	7-8
	Overwhelming Pain	9-10

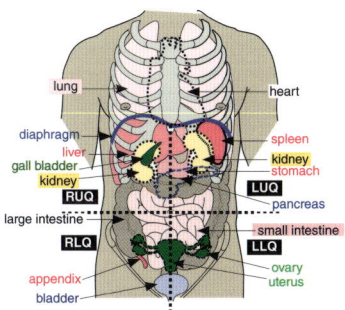

Abdominal Pain—Common Causes

- **Epigastric:** AMI, gastroenteritis, ulcer, esophageal disease, heartburn
- **LUQ:** Gastritis, pancreatitis, AMI, pneumonia
- **LLQ:** Ruptured ectopic pregnancy, ovarian cyst, PID, kidney stones, diverticulitis, enteritis, abdominal abscess
- **RLQ:** Appendicitis, ruptured ectopic pregnancy, enteritis, diverticulitis, PID, ovarian cyst, kidney stones, abdominal abscess, strangulated hernia
- **RUQ:** Gallstones, hepatitis, liver disease, pancreatitis, appendicitis, perforated duodenal ulcer, AMI, pneumonia
- **Midline:** Bladder infection, aortic aneurysm, uterine disease, intestinal disease, early appendicitis
- **Diffuse Pain:** Pancreatitis, peritonitis, appendicitis, gastroenteritis, dissecting or rupturing aortic aneurysm, diabetes, ischemic bowel, sickle cell crisis

Abdominal Pain

Hx—N/V (color/quality of emesis), bowel movements, dysuria, menstrual history, fever, **postural hypotension**, referred shoulder pain? Consider ectopic pregnancy. Genitourinary, vaginal, or rectal bleeding/discharge? Examine all 4 quadrants: **abdominal tenderness, guarding, rigidity**, bowel tones present? Distension, pulsatile mass? Vitals (sitting and supine), Chemstrip®. Peripheral pulses equal?

Treatment—Position of comfort and NPO. Consider pulse oximetry. O_2, IV (adjusted to vitals), consider ECG for epigastric pain.

Cautions—Consider aortic aneurysm, ectopic pregnancy, DKA. Epigastric abdominal pain may be cardiac.

Consider:

- **Abdominal Aortic Aneurysm:** Severe abdominal pain, pulsatile mass, hypotension
- **Acute MI:** Chest "pressure" or epigastric pain radiating to left arm or jaw; diaphoresis, N/V, SOB, pallor, dysrhythmias
- **Appendicitis:** N/V, RLQ or periumbilical pain, fever, shock
- **Bowel Obstruction:** N/V (fecal odor), localized pain
- **Cholecystitis:** Acute onset RUQ pain and tenderness (may be referred to right shoulder/scapula)—may be related to high-fat meal; N/V, anorexia, fever.
- **Ectopic Pregnancy:** Missed period, pelvic pain, abnormal vaginal bleeding, dizziness
- **Food Poisoning:** N/V, diffuse abdominal pain and cramping, diarrhea, fever, weakness, dizziness. Severe symptom: paralysis
- **Hepatic Failure:** Jaundice, confusion/coma, edema, bleeding and bruising, renal failure, Fv, anorexia, dehydration
- **Kidney Stone:** Colicky severe flank pain, hematuria, N/V
- **Pancreatitis:** Severe, "sharp" or "twisting" epigastric or LUQ pain radiating to back; N/V, distention, fever, shock
- **Ulcer:** "Burning," epigastric pain, N/V, possible hematemesis

■ Abuse

Intentional Trauma

Remove patient from the environment. Report possible abuse to police, ED staff, and child welfare office. Call for police assistance if needed to remove patient from the scene. **Do not confront the alleged abuser.** Document your findings and any statements made by child, parent, or others. Provide medical care as needed. If sexual abuse, do not allow patient to wash.

Child Maltreatment

Hx—Any unusual MOI, or one that does not match the child's injury or illness. Parents may accuse the child of hurting themself or may be vague or contradictory in providing Hx. There may be a delay in seeking medical care. **The child may not cling to mother.** Fx in any child < 2 yo; **multiple injuries in various stages of healing** or on many parts of the body; obvious cigarette burns or wire marks; **malnutrition**; insect infestation, chronic skin infection, or unkempt patient.

Intimate Partner Violence

Repeated ED visits, with injuries becoming more severe with each visit; **minimizing the seriousness** or frequency of the injuries; seeking treatment ≥ 1 day after the injury; **injuries that are not likely to have been caused by the incident reported**; overprotective significant other who does not allow the patient to be alone with the healthcare professional; **fractures in different stages of healing** according to radiographic findings; history of child abuse to patient or partner.

Medical

Older Adult Maltreatment

Fractures or bruises at various stages of healing; unexplained bruises or cigarette burns on the torso or extremities; soft-tissue injuries from signs of restraint use; head injuries; malnourishment, listlessness, dehydration unexplained; **poor hygiene**, inappropriate clothing; decubitus ulcer, **urine and feces on body and clothing**; unusual interaction between caregiver and patient.

■ Altered Mental Status

Safety: Consider personal and crew safety

Present History: Onset, witnessed, previous episode, trauma, fever, headache, chest pain, pill bottles, syringes, gas odor, street drugs?

Past History: Alcoholism, seizures, diabetes, thyroid condition, renal condition, TIA or CVA, HTN, medications, pregnancy, Alzheimer disease, COPD, psychiatric conditions, previous suicide attempt?

Medications: New medications, insulin or oral hypoglycemic, pill count and date filled, last oral intake?

Physical Examination:

- Vital signs
- General appearance, trauma, speech pattern, incontinent of urine
- Airway: Gag reflex, tongue lacerations
- Breathing: Breath odor, lung sounds, respiratory rate, oxygen saturation
- Circulation: Heart rate, regular/irregular
- Disability: Moves all extremities, alert/oriented, blood glucose
- Eyes: Deviation, pupils (size, reactive), nystagmus
- Skin: Rashes, needle tracks, cutting, scars

AEIOU TIPS Mnemonic for Coma			
A	Alcohol/Acidosis	T	Trauma/Tumors/Temp
E	Epilepsy	I	Infection
I	Insulin/Infection	P	Psychiatric/Poisoning
O	Opiates/Overdose	S	Subdural/Stroke
U	Uremia/Underdose			

■ Psychiatric Emergencies

Hx—History of recent crisis? Emotional trauma, suicidal, changes in behavior, drug/alcohol abuse? Toxins, head injury, diabetes, seizure disorder, sepsis or other illness? Ask about suicidal feelings, intent; does patient have a plan? Make judgement about whether patient will act on plan. **Vitals with pupil signs, mental status, oriented? Any odor on breath? MedicAlert® tags? Any signs of trauma? Make sure scene is safe—Protect Yourself!**

Psychiatric Signs/Symptoms:

- Mood disorders: Depression, mania, suicide ideation, anxiety
- Thought disorders: Delusions, hallucinations, pressured speech, racing thoughts, grandiose or paranoid ideation

Contact OLMC or psychiatric hospital. ABCs, restrain patient as needed. If patient is suicidal do not leave alone. Remove dangerous objects (weapons, pills, etc). Transport in calm, quiet manner, if possible. Consider: O_2, IV, check blood sugar. If low, consider glucose, PO or IV.

Cautions—Always suspect hypoglycemia, and look for other medical causes: ETOH, drugs, sepsis, CVA, hypoxia, CNS infection—may mimic psychiatric illness. Never assume patient's condition is purely psychiatric.

Medical

■ Respiratory Distress

Disease	Lung Sounds	Other S/Sx; Notes
Asthma	Wheezing, crackles	Hx allergies
Bronchitis	Wheezing, crackles	Recent respiratory tract infection, smoker
Heart failure	Crackles, wheezes	Pedal edema, history HF, patient takes beta-blocker, Lasix
Emphysema (COPD)	Wheezing, rhonchi	Smoker; barrel chest; patient takes CombiVent, O_2
Foreign body obstruction	Stridor, wheezing	Heard best right over the site of the obstruction
Pneumonia	Scattered crackles, wheezing	Fever; brown, green, or yellow sputum; dehydration
Pneumothorax	Decreased on one side	Deviated trachea (late); hyperresonant percussion

NOTE: When in doubt about the cause of the patient's respiratory distress, give oxygen. Hyperventilation of unknown origin can be shock, sepsis, stroke, drug overdose

Go to next page

Hx—Onset of event: was it slow or fast? Fever? Cough? Is cough productive? Recent respiratory infection? Does patient smoke (how much)? Record patient's medications. **Assess severity of dyspnea** (mild, moderate, severe) and tidal volume. **Single-word sentences? Is cyanosis present?** Level of consciousness? Accessory muscle use? Agitation? Lung sounds: any wheezing, crackles, rhonchi, diminished sounds? Vitals? Pulse oximetry, EtCO$_2$? **Is patient exhausted? Candidate for intubation?** Upper airway obstruction (stridor, hoarseness, drooling, coughing)? Chest pain? Itching, hives? Numbness of mouth and hands? Signs of HF: JVD, wet lung sounds (crackles), peripheral edema?

Treatment:

- **General Treatment:** Position of comfort (usually upright). Give O$_2$ as needed. **Be prepared to assist ventilations.** Monitor ECG, vitals. Start IV.

  Cautions—High-flow O$_2$ can depress respirations in a patient with COPD. Prepare to assist respirations.

- **Anaphylaxis**: See *Allergic Reaction* on the next page.
- **Asthma:**
  - ❏ **ADULT:** Consider nebulized bronchodilator, and/or epinephrine 1 mg/mL (1:1000) IM (0.3 mg–0.5 mg). If asthma is moderate-to-severe and not improving with treatment, administer dexamethasone 10 mg IV/IO/IM/PO
  - ❏ **INFANT/CHILDREN:** Administer nebulized bronchodilator and/or epinephrine 1 mg/mL (1:1000) IM (max dose 0.5 mg). If asthma is moderate-to-severe and not improving with treatment, consider dexamethasone 0.6 mg/kg IV/IO/IM/PO, up to 10 mg.
- **COPD**: Consider nebulized bronchodilator and CPAP.
- **Pulmonary Edema**: Consider nebulized bronchodilator, CPAP, and sublingual nitroglycerin.
- **Tension Pneumothorax**: Contact OLMC. Lift occlusive dressing. **Rapid transport**.

Medical

■ Asthma Severity Assessment

Asthma Severity Assessment Guide			
	MILD	**MODERATE**	**SEVERE**
Short of breath	Walking	Talking	At rest
Able to speak	In sentences	In phrases	In words
Heart rate	< 100	100 - 120	> 120
Respiratory rate	Elevated	Elevated	> 30
Lung sound	End expiratory wheezing	Full expiratory wheezes	Wheezes both phases
Accessory muscle use	Not usually	Common	Usually
Alertness	Possible agitated	Usually agitated	Usually agitated
$EtCO_2$	20 - 30	30 - 40	> 40

■ Allergic Reaction—Anaphylaxis

Hx—Mild reaction (local swelling only); or serious systemic reaction (hives, **pallor, bronchospasm, wheezing, upper airway obstruction** with **stridor**, swelling of throat, **hypotension**)? **(If cardiac arrest, treat per ACLS.)**

Treatment—If bee sting, remove stinger (scrape, do not squeeze).
- For mild local reaction: Wash area, apply cold pack.
- For serious reaction: Move directly to EpiPen® 0.3 mg autoinjector, IM (lateral thigh is best site); secure airway, ventilate, O_2; large-bore IV, titrate to BP > 90; ECG;

Peds—EpiPen Jr® 0.15 mg autoinjector

Cautions—Epinephrine may cause arrhythmias or angina.

◼ Shock

Hx—Onset? Associated symptoms: hives, edema, thirst, weakness, dyspnea, chest pain, dizziness when upright, abdominal pain? **Trauma?** Bloody vomitus or stools? Delayed capillary refill? Tachypnea? Syncope? N/V? **Mental status: confusion, restlessness?** Tachycardia, hypotension? **Skin: pale, sweaty, cool.** Signs of pump failure: JVD while upright, crackles, peripheral edema.

Treatment—Stop hemorrhage if any, apply direct pressure to wound. Consider hemostatic dressing or tourniquet. Place patient supine, O_2 high flow, assist ventilations as needed. **Do not delay transport to start IV** (consider intraosseous infusion if unable to start IV). Give IV fluid challenge. Prevent heat loss. Try to determine the type of shock (hypovolemic, cardiogenic, anaphylactic, septic, neurogenic, etc.). **If trauma, enter patient in Trauma System.** Assess lung sounds. Monitor ECG, O_2 saturation, vitals, level of consciousness.

Cautions—Check lung sounds for crackles before giving IV fluids.

◼ Endocrine

Hyperglycemia

Hx—Slow onset, excessive urination, thirst. When was insulin last taken? Abdominal cramps, N/V? Mental status, high glucose level on strip test, skin signs, dehydration? Respirations: deep and rapid? Breath odor: acetone, fruity?

Secure airway; get vital signs, give O_2, large-bore IV fluid challenge (isotonic crystalloid solution, NS or LR). Monitor ECG.

Hypoglycemia/Insulin Shock

Hx—Sudden onset, low blood glucose level on CBG test. Last insulin dose? Last meal? Mental status? Diaphoresis, H/A, blurred vision, dizziness, tachycardia, tremors, seizures?

Support ABCs, give O_2, take vital signs, start IV fluids. Give 50 mL $D_{50}W$ PO/NG/IV, if patient comatose (perform CBG before and after). Consider glucagon IM if IV not possible. **Do not give oral glucose if airway is compromised.**

Caution: Hypoglycemia can mimic a stroke or intoxication. Seizures, coma, and confusion are common symptoms. When in doubt about the diagnosis, give glucose IV or PO.

Hypoglycemia Versus Hyperglycemia

	Hypoglycemia (Insulin Shock)	Hyperglycemia (Ketoacidosis)
Incidence	More common	Less common
Blood sugar	Low (≤ 80 mg/dL)	High (≥ 180 mg/dL)
Onset	Rapid (minutes)	Gradual (days)
Skin	Moist, pale	Dry, warm
Respirations	Normal	Deep or rapid
Pulse	Normal or fast	Rapid, weak
Blood pressure	Normal or high	Normal or low
Breath odor	Normal	Ketone/acetone odor
Seizures	Common	Uncommon
Dehydration	No	Yes
Urine output	Normal	Excessive
Thirst	Normal	Very thirsty
Mental status	Disoriented, coma	Awake, weak, tired
Treatment	Glucose IV or PO	IV fluids, insulin, K^+
Recovery	Rapid (minutes)	Gradual (days)

NOTE: When in doubt about the diagnosis, give glucose IV or PO.

Infectious Diseases

Infectious Diseases of Special Concern

Disease	Spread by	Risk to You
AIDS/HIV	IV/sex/blood products	↓ Immune function, pneumonias, cancer
Anthrax	*Cutaneous:* contact with skin lesions	Infection = 25% mortality, but much lower if treated
	Ingestion: eating contaminated meat	Infection = high mortality, unless treated with antibiotics
	Pulmonary: inhaled spores	Infection = 95% mortality, but much lower if treated
Chickenpox	Airborne/skin contact	Fever, itchy rash, blisters, shingles
Clostridium difficile	Secretions/excretions Antibiotic use	Diarrhea, nausea, shock
COVID-19	Airborne	Primarily respiratory illness, but can affect multiple body systems
Ebola	Airborne/blood	Viral hemorrhagic fever
Hepatitis A*	Fecal-oral	Acute hepatitis, jaundice
Hepatitis B*	IV/sex/birth/blood	Acute and chronic hepatitis, cirrhosis, liver cancer
Hepatitis C	Blood	Chronic hepatitis, cirrhosis, liver cancer
Hepatitis D	IV/sex/birth	Chronic liver disease
Hepatitis E	Fecal-oral	↑ Mortality to pregnant women and fetus
Herpes	Skin contact	Skin lesions, shingles
Influenza	Droplet/airborne	Fever, pneumonia, prostration

Go to next page

Medical

Infectious Diseases of Special Concern

Disease	Spread by	Risk to You
MRSA	Secretions/excretions Hand to nose	Ulceration, tissue destruction
Meningitis*	Nasal secretions	Low risk to rescuer
Monkey Pox	Airborne/skin contact/sex	Fever
Norovirus	Fecal-oral Hand to mouth	Diarrhea, nausea, vomiting
Tuberculosis	Sputum/cough/airborne	Cough, weight loss, lung damage

*Get vaccinated against hepatitis A, B, and meningitis A, C, W, Y.

Standard Precautions/BSI

- Wear gloves for all patient contacts and for all contacts with body fluids.
- Wash hands before and after patient contact.
- Place a mask on patients who are coughing or sneezing.
- Place a mask on yourself.
- Wear eye shields or goggles for all patient contacts
- Wear gowns when needed.
- Wear utility gloves for cleaning equipment.
- Do not recap, cut, or bend needles.

CAUTION: Report every exposure and get immediate treatment!

COVID/Influenza-like Illness

- Surgical mask on patient ASAP.
- Limit providers/equipment.
- Providers wear N95 masks for transport and aerosol-generating procedures (AGPs)

For use with patients with known or suspected high-risk infections (i.e., Ebola, SARS, MERS)

Preparation:

- PPE should be available for isolation precautions recommended for the infection encountered (airborne, contact, and droplet). This may require N-95 masks, Tyvek® suits, boots, duct tape to seal seams, etc.
- EMS personnel should be trained and regularly practice donning and doffing PPE.
- Consider coordinating with local HazMat for training and response.
- Vehicles should be outfitted with isolation materials and carry appropriate cleaning and decontamination supplies recommended for known infectious agents.
- EMS should have Public Health contact information (see *Phone Numbers*).

Response:

- Only properly equipped and trained responders should be dispatched.
- Minimize equipment carried in to scene.
- One provider in appropriate PPE should enter scene to interview patient. A second provider in PPE should be available in case initial provider requires immediate assistance.
- Other providers on scene should act as trained observers, monitoring PPE donning and activities to ensure consistency with training and best practices.
- The patient should be provided with a surgical mask to wear prior to the provider moving closer than 6 feet. If the patient is vomiting, they should be provided with an emesis bag to contain any vomitus. If the patient's clothes are soiled, the patient should be provided with a protective suit to don prior to transport (if possible).

Go to next page

Medical

- Any family members or other individuals on scene should be separated from the patient and asked to remain in a safe location on scene until consult can be made with Public Health authorities.

Discovery of High-Risk Patient After Responding:

- If a responder encounters a patient they suspect may have a high-risk biological condition or disease, they should immediately contact the dispatch center to request an appropriate response.
- To avoid contamination, the crew should not leave the scene or reenter their response vehicles.

Transport:

- If the patient is stable and ambulatory, they should be walked to the ambulance by the provider making initial contact, with advance notice to any providers outside so there is a clear path to the ambulance. If extraction is required, then the minimum number of personnel in appropriate PPE should be utilized to safely move the patient.
- The ambulance patient compartment should be isolated from the cab and the driver donned in appropriate PPE. If the patient can be properly cared for by a single provider, then the crew should be limited to one care provider and one driver.
- Destination hospital should be notified by telephone prior to arrival and agreed upon transfer location determined.

Decontamination:

- Public Health authorities should be notified of the scene location to arrange for decon of the premises.
- Crew members and transport vehicle should be decontaminated following recommended disease specific procedures.

Surveillance:

- Any crew members with exposure or patient contact should be followed by department occupational safety and health provider.
- Appropriate testing, prophylaxis, and quarantine should be utilized following disease-specific recommendations.

Neurologic

■ Stroke

EMS Assessment and Treatment

- Support ABCs, give O$_2$, check glucose level.
- Perform stroke assessment (see *LAPSS* or *CPSS*, after *Stroke*).
- Establish onset of symptoms.
- **Rapid transport to stroke center** (bring family member).
- Notify hospital: "stroke alert."

Immediate Assessment and Stabilization

- Activate stroke team.
- Check ABCs, vital signs; give O$_2$ if hypoxemic.
- Start IV fluids; get blood samples; 12-lead ECG.
- Check blood glucose level: correct hypoglycemia/hyperglycemia.
- Perform general neurologic screening assessment.
- Initiate emergency CT scan or MRI of brain.

Immediate Neurologic Assessment by Stroke Team

- Review patient history.
- Establish onset of symptoms.
- Perform neurologic examination (NIH Stroke Scale or Canadian Neurologic Scale).

■ Los Angeles Prehospital Stroke Screen (LAPSS)

Screening Criteria:

1. Age older than 45 years ❑ Yes ❑ No
2. No prior history of seizure disorder ❑ Yes ❑ No
3. New neurologic symptoms in last 24 hours ❑ Yes ❑ No
4. Patient was ambulatory before event ❑ Yes ❑ No
5. Blood glucose level of 60–400 mg/dL ❑ Yes ❑ No
6. Examination (below) reveals only unilateral weakness ❑ Yes ❑ No

Examination: Look for Obvious Asymmetry			
	Normal	Right	Left
Facial smile/grimace	❑	Droop ❑	Droop ❑
Grip	❑	Weak grip ❑	Weak grip ❑
		No grip ❑	No grip ❑
Arm weakness	❑	Drifts down ❑	Drifts down ❑
		Falls rapidly ❑	Falls rapidly ❑

7. If "yes" to all items above, the LAPSS screening criteria are met:
   Notify receiving hospital with "code stroke."

NOTE: The patient may still be experiencing a stroke even if LAPSS criteria are not met.

■ LVO: Large Vessel Occlusion

- ■ Considered one of the most severe types of stroke with obstruction of large proximal cerebral artery (high mortality, poor outcomes).

S/S: Sudden loss of balance/coordination, facial drooping, blurred vision, slurred speech, weakness in one arm, eye deviation (does patient partially look to one side or have a forced eye deviation?), denial/neglect (does patient appear to be ignoring one side of their own body when stimulus is applied?).

- ■ Occlusion of posterior large vessels occur in 20% of all ischemic strokes and can be identified by assessing **dizziness, drowsiness, dysarthria, diplopia** and **dysphagia**. Observe for facial palsy, arm weakness, speech changes, eye deviation, and denial/neglect.

Advanced Notification by EMS:

- ■ Notify hospital with exact time of onset.
- ■ Place two large-bore IVs for facilitation of advanced imaging. Also include next of kin contact information for additional questions/information.
- ■ Advanced notification facilitates activation of stroke team, CT scanners, pharmacy, and preparation for your arrival.

■ Cincinnati Prehospital Stroke Scale (CPSS)

Symptoms	Normal	Abnormal
Facial droop	Both sides of face move equally	One side of face does not move as well as other side
Arm drift	Both arms move equally or not at all	One arm drifts compared with the other
Speech	Patient uses correct words with no slurring	Slurred or inappropriate words or mute

NOTE: Any abnormal finding suggests potential stroke.

Neurologic

Seizures

Consider epilepsy, hypoxia, CVA, cardiac origin, ETOH/drug withdrawal, hypoglycemia.

Hx—Onset, length of seizure, type? Previous history? Seizure medications? Compliance? **Recent head trauma?** What was patient doing before seizure? Did patient fall? Bite tongue? Dysrhythmias? Incontinent? Is Sz drug-induced (antidepressant, cocaine)? MedicAlert®? Level of consciousness, head or oral trauma? Focal neurologic signs? H/A? Respiratory status? **Treatment for status epilepticus:** Keep airway open, consider NPA, O₂, suction, IV, check blood glucose, consider IV glucose. Transport on side, monitor ECG, vitals.

Cautions—Restrain patient only to prevent injury—protect patient's head. Do not force anything into the mouth. Always check for a pulse after a seizure stops. Most seizures are self-limiting, lasting less than 1–2 minutes.

Posturing

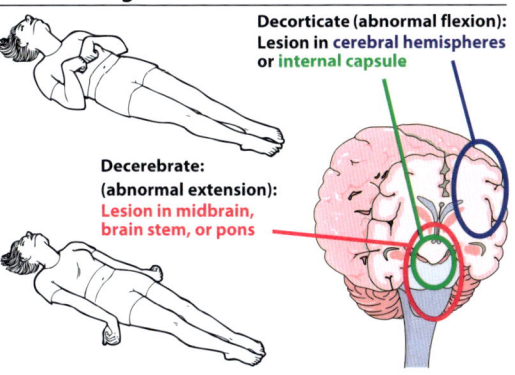

Decorticate (abnormal flexion): Lesion in cerebral hemispheres or internal capsule

Decerebrate: (abnormal extension): Lesion in midbrain, brain stem, or pons

Early signs of ↑ICP:

Change in LOC is the most important sign. Other S/S: restlessness, lethargy, confusion, headache, disorientation. VS changes may occur later: ↑BP, ↓HR, respiratory pattern changes. Seizures, pupillary changes are usually a late sign of ↑ICP.

Prolonged ↑ICP may result in herniation. Signs of herniation (pressure on the brain stem and surrounding area) are ↓LOC, decorticate or decerebrate posturing, and pupillary changes.

■ Cranial Nerves

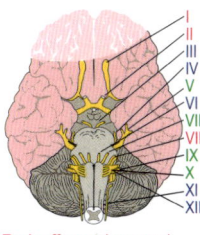

I	Olfactory (smell)
II	Optic (sight, visual acuity/fields, fundus)
III	Oculomotor (pupil constriction, eye movement)
IV	Trochlear (downward, inward gaze)
V	Trigeminal (facial sensory, chewing)
VI	Abducens (lateral eye movement)
VII	Facial (taste, frown, smile)
VIII	Accoustic (hearing, balance)
IX	Glossopharyngeal (throat, taste, gag, swallowing)
X	Vagus (larynx, voice, ↓HR)
XI	Spinal Accessory (shoulder shrug)
XII	Hypoglossal (tongue movement)

Red: afferent (sensory)
Blue: efferent (motor)
Green: both

Neurologic

■ Glasgow Coma Scale

NOTE: A score of 3 is considered a coma; ≤8 requires intubation and airway management.

INFANT		Eye Opening		CHILD/ADULT
	4	Spontaneously	Spontaneously	4
	3	To speech	To command	3
	2	To pain	To pain	2
_____	1	No response	No response	1 _____
		Best Verbal Response		
	5	Coos, babbles	Oriented	5
	4	Irritable cries	Confused	4
	3	Cries to pain	Inappropriate words	3
	2	Moans, grunts	Incomprehensible	2
_____	1	No response	No response	1 _____
		Best Motor Response		
	6	Spontaneous	Obeys commands	6
	5	Localizes pain	Localizes pain	5
	4	Withdraws from pain	Withdraws from pain	4
	3	Flexion (decorticate)	Flexion (decorticate)	3
	2	Extension (decerebrate)	Extension (decerebrate)	2
_____	1	No response	No response	1 _____
_____		= Total	Total =	_____

Go to next page

Interpretation of GCS:	
15:	Normal
13–14:	Minor injury to head
9–12:	Moderate injury to head
3–8:	Severe injury to head
4–7:	Coma may be present
3:	Deep coma or brain death

Pupil Gauge (in mm)

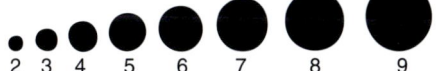

2 3 4 5 6 7 8 9

■ Concussion in Sports

On-Field Mental Status Evaluation

This mental status assessment is recommended for high school–age athletes and older. Any inability of the athlete to respond correctly to the questions below should be considered abnormal.

Orientation
What period/quarter/half are we in?
What stadium/field is this?
What city is this?
Who is the opposing team?
Who scored last?
What team did we play last?
Anterograde Amnesia
Ask the athlete to repeat the following words:
Girl, Dog, Green
Retrograde Amnesia
Ask the athlete the following:
Do you remember the hit?
What happened in the play prior to the hit?
What happened in the quarter/period prior to the hit?
What was the score of the game prior to the hit?
Concentration
Ask the athlete to do the following:
Repeat the days of the week backwards (starting with today)
Repeat the months of the year backward (starting with December)
Repeat these numbers backward 63 (36), 419 (914), 6294 (4926)
Word List Memory
Ask the athlete to repeat the three words from earlier:
Girl, Dog, Green

Reproduced from: "Heads Up: Brain Injury in Your Practice" tool kit developed by the Centers for Disease Control and Prevention (CDC).

No Return to Play

Any athlete who exhibits signs and symptoms of concussion should be removed from play and should not participate in games or practices until they have been evaluated and given permission by an appropriate health care provider. Research indicates that high school athletes with fewer than 15 minutes of on-field symptoms exhibited deficits on formal neuropsychological testing and re-emergence of active symptoms, lasting up to one week post-injury.[1]

[1]Lovell MR, Collins MW, Bradley J. Return to play following sports-related concussion. Clinics in Sports Medicine 2004;23(3):421-41.

Signs of Deteriorating Neurologic Function

An athlete should be taken to the emergency department if any of the following signs and/or symptoms are present:

- Headaches that worsen
- Seizures
- Focal neurologic signs
- Looks very drowsy or can't be awakened
- Repeated vomiting
- Slurred speech
- Can't recognize people or places
- Increasing confusion or irritability
- Weakness or numbness in arms or legs
- Neck pain
- Unusual behavior change
- Significant irritability
- Any loss of consciousness lasting over 30 seconds. (Brief loss of consciousness [under 30 seconds] should be taken seriously and the patient should be carefully monitored.)

Poisons and Overdoses

NOTE: This section is not a comprehensive list of all drugs, poisons, adverse effects, cautions, or treatments. Before administering any treatments, consult your poison center, the product label or insert, your protocols, and/or your online medical resource.

◼ Abbreviations Used in This Section

AKA—Common brands®™ and "street names"

SE—Common toxic side effects (green text)

RX—Prehospital care (blue text)

Cautions—Primary cautions (red text)

◼ Poisons

Acetaminophen • *Analgesic*

AKA—Tylenol®, APAP.

SE—There may be no symptoms, but acetaminophen is toxic to the liver. N/V, anorexia, RUQ pain, pallor, diaphoresis, agitation, fatigue, anxiety, rash, anemia.

RX—ABCs, O_2, IV, ECG, fluids for hypotension. Activated charcoal 1 g/kg PO or by NG tube, if given within 4 hours of ingestion. Acetylcysteine may be given in the ED.

Cautions—Other pain meds may contain acetaminophen! Do not exceed 4g/day in healthy adults, or 2g/day in patients with hepatic insufficiency or who consume more than 3 alcoholic drinks a day.

Stages of Acute Acetaminophen Overdose		
Stage	Post-Ingestion Time	Symptoms
1	0–24 hours	N/V, anorexia
2	24–72 hours	RUQ pain, ALT, AST, INR, bilirubin begins to elevate
3	72–96 hours	Peaking ALT, AST, INR, bilirubin, vomiting. Renal failure and pancreatitis may be present
4	>5 days	Resolve hepatoxicity or progress to multiple-organ failure, may be fatal

Acids   • *Caustics*

AKA—Rust remover, metal polish.

SE—Pain, GI tract chemical burns, lip burns, vomiting.

RX—Give milk or water, milk of magnesia, egg white, prevent aspiration. Transport patient in sitting position, if possible.

Cautions—Do not induce vomiting.

Alkalis   • *Caustics*

AKA—Drano®, drain and oven cleaners, bleach.

SE—Pain, GI tract chemical burns, lip burns, vomiting.

RX—Give milk or water, prevent aspiration. Transport patient in sitting position, if possible.

Cautions—Do not induce vomiting.

Amphetamines/Stimulants • *Stimulants*

AKA—Methamphetamine, "Speed," "Crank," "Black Beauties," "Crystal Meth," "Fire," "Bikers," "Uppers," "Ice."

SE—Anxiety, $\uparrow$ HR, arrhythmias, confusion, hallucinations, agitation, seizure, chronic fatigue, insomnia, rotting of gums and teeth, skin abscesses, rhabdomyolysis, N/V, H/A, CVA, HTN, hyperthermia, hypertension, delusions, aggression, paranoia, dilated pupils, toxic psychosis, suicidal ideation, respiratory arrest, depression.

RX—ABCs, O_2, ECG, IV fluids for hypotension. Activated charcoal 50–100 g orally. Rapid cooling to maintain normal body temperature. Benzodiazepine as adjunct.

Cautions—Restraints or other measures to protect patient and yourself from harm.

Antidepressants (TCA) • *Mood Elevators*

AKA—Norpramin®, doxepin, amitriptyline, Elavil®.

SE—Hypotension, PVCs, cardiac arrhythmias, QRS complex widening, seizures, coma, death, torsades de pointes.

RX—ABCs, O_2, IV, ECG, IV fluids, 1 mEq/kg $NaHCO_3$ IV, intubate and ventilate.

Cautions—Onset of coma and seizures can be sudden. Do not induce vomiting.

Aspirin • *Analgesic*

AKA—Bayer®, ASA, salicylates.

SE—GI bleeding, N/V, LUQ pain, pallor, diaphoresis, shock, tinnitus, $\uparrow$ RR.

RX—ABCs, O_2, IV, ECG, fluids for hypotension. Activated charcoal 1 g/kg PO.

Barbiturates/Sedatives · *Hypnotics*

AKA—Phenobarbital, "Barbs," "Downers," "GHB," "Benzodiazepines."

SE—Weakness, drowsiness, respiratory depression, hypoventilation, apnea, coma, hypotension, bradycardia, hypothermia, APE, death.

RX—ABCs, O_2, ventilate, IV fluids for hypotension, supportive therapy.

Cautions—Protect the patient's airway.

"Bath Salts" Psychoactive · *Stimulant*

AKA—"Legal high", "Plant food", "Jewelry cleaner", "Flakka", "Ivory Wave", "Cloud Nine", "Vanilla Sky", "Bliss", "Mad Cow", "Room Deodorizer"

SE—Agitation, tachycardia, HTN, HA, hyperthermia, diaphoresis, hallucinatins, euphoria, anxiety, panic attack, psychosis, blurry vision, insomnia, ringing/buzzing in ears, nightmares, depression, aggression, tremors, paranoia, suicidal thoughts, N&V, DIC, anemia, thrombocytopenia, hyponatremia, acidosis, MI, rhabdomyolsis, renal failure, seizures, death.

RX—ABCs, vitals, IV, EKG. Consider benzodiazepine for agitation, panic attack, seizures. Cool the hyperthermic patient.

Cautions—Restraints or other measures to protect the patient. Protect yourself from harm.

Benzodiazepines · *Sedative/Hypnotics*

AKA—Valium®, Xanax®, diazepam, midazolam.

SE—Sedation, weakness, dizziness, tachycardia, hypotension, hypothermia (↓ respirations with IV use).

RX—ABCs, monitor VS; flumazenil IV if no seizure history.

Cautions—Coma usually means some other substance or cause is also involved. OD is almost always in combination with other drugs. Protect the patient's airway.

β-Blockers • *β-Adrenergic Blocking Agents*

AKA—Atenolol, Inderal®, metoprolol.

SE—Hypotension, bradycardia, hypoglycemia, bronchospasm, heart blocks, pulmonary edema, seizures, AMS, tachycardia.

RX—ABCs, monitor VS, activated charcoal (if within 1 h of ingestion), glucagon (5–10 mg IV followed by infusion 1–5 mg/h in adults), atropine, pacing, pressors; ED may use IV lipid emulsions and/or high-dose insulin w/glucose.

Cautions—Bradycardia, HF, hypotension, dyspnea, dizziness, heart block, cardiogenic shock, cardiac arrest, fatigue, dizziness.

Calcium Channel Antagonists/ Blockers (CCBs) • *Antagonists/ Blocking Agents*

AKA—Diltiazem, verapamil, amlodipine, nifedipine.

SE—Hypotension, bradycardia, N/V, metabolic acidosis, hyperglycemia.

RX—ABCs, activated charcoal, IV calcium chloride or gluconate, IV glucagon, pressors/catecholamines, pacing; ED may use IV lipid emulsions and/or high-dose insulin w/glucose.

Cautions—May require large doses of calcium, atropine loses effectiveness later in toxic doses.

Carbon Monoxide • *Odorless Toxic Gas*

Causes—Any source of incomplete combustion, such as car exhaust, fire suppression, and stoves.

SE—H/A, dizziness, DOE, fatigue, tachycardia, visual disturbances, hallucinations, cherry red skin color, ↓ respirations, N/V, cyanosis, altered mental status, coma, blindness, hearing loss, convulsions.

RX—Remove patient from toxic environment, ABCs, 100% O_2 (check blood glucose), transport. Hyperbaric treatment in severe cases.

Cautions—O_2 saturation monitor can give false high reading with CO exposure.

WARNING: Protect yourself from exposure!

Cardiac Glycosides • *Digoxin*

AKA—Digoxin, digitoxin (not available in U.S.).

SE—N/V, abdominal pain, bradycardia, heart blocks, hyperkalemia, AMS, weakness.

RX—ABCs, activated charcoal, atropine, DigiFab (dose per serum drug level and weight based on Poison Control recommendation), pacing, lidocaine for ventricular arrhythmias.

Cautions—Peak effects take 6–12 h, often asymptomatic initially, serum drug levels are valuable in dx/tx (therapeutic digoxin level 0.5–2 ng/mL, digitoxin 10–30 ng/mL).

Cocaine/Crack Cocaine • *Stimulant/Anesthetic*

AKA—"Coke," "Snow," "Flake," "Candy," "Dust," "Powder," "Charlie."

SE—H/A, N/V, ↓ RR, respiratory arrest, agitation, ↑ HR, arrhythmias, chest pain, vasoconstriction, AMI, HTN, seizure, vertigo, euphoria, hyperthermia, confusion, hallucinations, delirium, rhabdomyolysis, depression, tremors, coma, dilated pupils, bradycardia, death, APE with IV use.

RX—ABCs, O_2, IV, ET intubation. Consider benzodiazepine for seizures, lidocaine for PVCs, nitrates and phentolamine for AMI. Control HTN. Monitor VS and core temperature: cool patient if hyperthermic. Minimize sensory stimulation. Consider activated charcoal for oral cocaine ingestion.

Cautions—Restraints or other measures to protect patient and yourself from harm. A "Speedball" is cocaine and heroin. Do not give β-blockers.

Ecstasy/MDMA • *Stimulant/Hallucinogen*

AKA—"XTC," "X," "Molly," "Lovers Speed," "Clarity," "Adam," "Empathy."

SE—Date rape, rape drug. Euphoria, hallucinations, agitation, teeth grinding (use of pacifiers), nausea, hyperthermia, sweating, HTN, tachycardia, renal and heart failure, dilated pupils, seizures, rhabdomyolysis, DIC, APE, CVA, coma, electrolyte imbalance, death.

RX—ABCs, O_2, VS, ECG, IV, cool patient if hyperthermic, intubate if unconscious, benzodiazepine for seizures and bicarbonate for myoglobinuria.

Cautions—Do not give β-blockers.

GHB (Gamma hydroxybutyrate), BD (1,4-Butanediol), and GBL (Gamma-butyrolactone) • *Depressants/Sedatives*

AKA—GHB: "Gib," "Liquid Ecstasy," "Nitro," "Soap." BD: "Serenity," "Revitalize Plus," "Thunder Nectar." GBL: "Blue Nitro," "GH Revitalizer," "Gamma G."

SE—Feeling affectionate, happy, euphoria, sedation, dizziness, seizures, N/V, loss of gag reflex, somnolence, hallucinations, weakness, LOC, coma, bradycardia, apnea, respiratory arrest, death.

RX—ABCs, manage airway, ventilate.

Cautions—A common "date rape" drug.

Hydrocarbons • *Fuels, Oils*

AKA—Gasoline, oil, petroleum products.

SE—Breath odor, SOB, seizures, acute pulmonary edema, coma, bronchospasm.

RX—ABCs, O_2, gastric lavage.

Cautions—Do not induce vomiting.

Jimson Weed (*Datura stramonium*) • *Hallucinogen*

AKA—"Thorn Apple," "Angel's Trumpet," "Devils Trumpet," "Stinkweed," "Locoweed," "Ditch Weed," "Mad Hatter."

SE—Euphoria, hallucinations, delirium, agitation, confusion, blurred vision, dilated pupils, thirst, dry mucous membranes, hyperthermia, dysphasia, dysphagia, tachycardia, coma, respiratory arrest, urinary retention, seizures.

RX—ABCs, cool patient, IV, sedation, calm and reassure the patient. Restraints or other measures to protect patient and yourself from harm.

Cautions—Combative behavior; plant contains dangerous chemicals such as atropine and scopolamine that can cause serious side effects, including death.

Khat (*Catha edulis*) • *Stimulant*

AKA—"Chat," "Kat," "Abyssinian Tea," "Oat," "African Salad," "Catha."

SE—Insomnia, hyperactivity, euphoria, hallucinations, tachycardia, hypertension, hypermanic state, paranoia, anger, delusions of grandeur, irritability, extreme thirst, constipation, dilated pupils.

RX—ABCs, IV, sedation, calm and reassure the patient. Restraints or other measures to protect patient and yourself from harm.

Cautions—Cardiac complication: MI; bleeding in the brain, chemical hepatitis, aggressive behavior, depression, severe migraines.

LSD (Lysergic Acid Diethylamide) • *Hallucinogen*

AKA—"Boomers," "Acid," "Hits," "Sugar Cubes," "Trips," "Yellow Sunshine."

SE—Tachycardia, HTN, hyperthermia, profuse perspiration, gooseflesh, dilated pupils, paranoia, hallucinations, delusions, panic reactions, and tremors. Flashbacks are an unpredictable and dangerous side effect that may occur days to months after use of drug.

RX—ABCs, cool patient, sedation, calm and reassure patient. Restraints or other measures to protect patient and yourself from harm.

Cautions—Watch for flashbacks with dangerous side effects, panic attacks.

Opiates • *Narcotic Analgesic*

AKA—Dilaudid®, heroin, morphine, codeine, fentanyl, methadone, oxycodone.

SE—↓ Respirations, apnea, ↓ BP, coma, bradycardia, pinpoint pupils, vomiting, diaphoresis, depressed mental status, cold/clammy skin, confusion, delirium, disorientation, seizures, death.

RX—ABCs, O_2, ventilate, intubate, IV fluids for hypotension, naloxone 2 mg IV/IO, IM, SC, ET, IL.

Cautions—Consider other concurrent overdoses.

Organophosphates • *Insecticides*

AKA—Malathion®, Diazinon®, Dibrom®.

SE—SLUDGE (Salivation, Lacrimation, Urination, Defecation, GI distress, Emesis), pinpoint pupils, weakness, bradycardia, sweating, N/V, diarrhea, dyspnea, tremors, confusion.

RX—Decontaminate patient, ABCs. O_2, atropine 1–5 mg IV/IO, IM. Double doses every 5 min until SLUDGE goes away. Start at 2 mg IV/IO, IM for moderate signs and symptoms. After initial treatment with atropine, other medications used to treat organophosphate poisonings are pralidoxime (2-PAM) and benzodiazepines (e.g., diazepam).

Peds—*0.05 mg/kg, every 5 min, until vital signs improve.*

Cautions—Protect yourself first! Do not become contaminated.

PCP—Phencyclidine • *Hallucinogen*

AKA—"Peace Pill," "Angel Dust," "Hog," "Ozone," "Rocket Fuel," "Crystal."

SE—Nystagmus, disorientation, HTN, hallucinations, distorted perception of sounds, severe agitation, violent behavior, coma, can succumb to pulmonary aspiration and cardiovascular collapse, catatonia, sedation, paralysis, stupor, mania, tachycardia, dilated pupils, status epilepticus.

RX—ABCs, O_2, vitals, IV, ECG. Activated charcoal if drug has been taken by mouth. Consider benzodiazepines or antipsychotics (e.g., haloperidol).

Cautions—Protect yourself against the violent patient. Examine patient for trauma that may have occurred due to anesthetic effect of PCP.

Psilocybin Mushrooms • *Hallucinogen*

AKA—"LSD," "Magic Mushrooms."

SE—Anxiety, panic, N/V, euphoria, disorientation, drowsiness, muscle weakness or relaxation, lack of coordination, dilated pupils, vivid visual and auditory hallucinations, synesthesia.

RX—Calm and reassure the patient. Be supportive, decrease sensory and emotional stimuli.

Cautions—Watch for violent and unexpected behavior. Restraints or other measures to protect the patient and yourself from harm. Risk of poisoning from mushrooms that were not psilocybin mushroom.

Salicylates

AKA—Aspirin, also contained in topical analgesics, liniments, antidiarrheal agents.

SE—Tachypnea, tinnitus, dizziness, deafness, hyperthermia, AMS, N/V, abdominal pain, GI bleeds, pulmonary edema, liver/kidney failure.

RX—ABCs, activated charcoal, replace potassium, monitor fluid volume status, alkalinize urine to reduce salicylate level.

Cautions—No antidote for salicylate poisoning, may require repeated doses of activated charcoal, hemodialysis may be needed.

SSRIs (and Noncyclic Antidepressants)   • *Antidepressants*

AKA—Fluoxetine, paroxetine, sertraline.

SE—Sedation, ataxia, dizziness, AMS, N/V, diarrhea, H/A, restlessness, shivering, diaphoresis, hypotension, QTc prolongation, muscle rigidity, tremors, seizures.

RX—ABCs, activated charcoal if needed, fluids for hypotension, IV benzodiazepines for seizures.

Cautions—SSRIs are relatively safe, toxicity is limited, few tests are widely available to aid in diagnosis/management of SSRI toxicity.

Toxic Alcohols

AKA—Ethylene glycol, methanol (found in antifreeze, windshield washer fluid).

SE—Ethylene glycol: ataxia, slurred speech, AMS, may have N/V, and then, after 4–12 hours, seizures, cerebral edema, coma. Methanol: classic ethanol intoxication s/s initially, may have N/V. Later: visual disturbances, blindness, AMS, seizures, hypotension, death.

RX—ABCs, ED may use gastric lavage, administer ethanol or fomepizole as antidotes to block metabolism and increase elimination. Hemodialysis may be needed.

Cautions—Protect the airway, consider intubation. Support ventilation, acute cardiac and renal symptoms.

Tranquilizers (Major) • *Antipsychotics*

AKA—Xanax®, Valium®, Ativan®, Klonopin®

SE—Drowsiness, dizziness, seizures, dystonias, respiratory depression, sluggishness, fatigue, hypotension.

RX—ABCs, O_2, vitals, ECG. IV fluids for hypotension. Consider intubation for the unconscious patient.

Cautions—Protect the patient's airway. Xanax not approved for anyone <18 yo.

Tricyclic Antidepressants (TCAs) • *Antidepressants*

AKA—Amitriptyline, doxepin, imipramine, nortriptyline.

SE—Dry mouth/skin, dilated pupils, seizures, delirium, agitation, hallucinations, tremors, hyperthermia, QRS widening, hypotension.

RX—ABCs, IV bicarbonate for ventricular arrhythmias or refractory hypotension, IV benzodiazapines for seizures, fluids or pressors for hypotension.

Cautions—TCAs are highly toxic, prescribed as last-resort antidepressants. Toxic dose is 10–20 mg/kg. Treat all overdoses as potentially life threatening. Protect the airway, consider intubation. Support ventilation, acute cardiac and renal symptoms.

Major Toxidromes

Toxidrome	Drug Examples	Signs and Symptoms	Antidotes
Stimulant	Amphetamine, methamphetamine, cocaine, diet aids, nasal decongestants	Restlessness, agitation, incessant talking, insomnia, anorexia; dilated pupils, tachycardia; diaphoresis, hyperthermia, tachypnea, hypertension or hypotension; paranoia, seizures, cardiac arrest	Benzodiazepine
Narcotic (opiate and opioid)	Heroin, opium, morphine, hydromorphone, (Dilaudid®), fentanyl, oxycodone–aspirin combination (Percodan®), methadone	Constricted (pinpoint) pupils, marked respiratory depression; needle tracks in IV abusers; drowsiness, stupor, coma, depressed mental status	Naloxone, nalmefene, naltrexone
Sympathomimetic	Pseudoephedrine, phenylephrine, phenylpropanolamine, amphetamine, cocaine and methamphetamine	Hypertension, tachycardia, dilated pupils (mydriasis), agitation and seizures, hyperthermia, diaphoresis	Benzodiazepine

Go to next page

Poisons

Toxidrome	Drug Examples	Signs and Symptoms	Antidotes
Sedative and hypnotic	Phenobarbital, diazepam (Valium®), thiopental, zolpidem tartrate (Ambien®), secobarbital	Drowsiness, disinhibition, ataxia, slurred speech, mental confusion, respiratory depression, progressive CNS depression, hypotension, hypothermia	None
Cholinergic (Anti-cholinesterase)	Diazinon, orthene; sarin, tabun, VX (nerve agents)	Increased salivation, lacrimation, GI distress, diarrhea, respiratory depression, apnea, seizures, coma	Atropine, pralidoxime
Anticholinergic	Atropine, scopolamine, antihistamines, antipsychotics, Jimson Weed	Dry, flushed skin; hyperthermia, dilated pupils, blurred vision, tachycardia; mild hallucinations, dramatic delirium	Physostigmine in ED

Trauma

Trauma Triage Chart

High Risk for Serious Injury

	All Patients	Age 0–9 yrs	Age 10–64 yrs	Age ≥65 yrs
Assessment:	■ Unable to follow commands (motor GCS <6) ■ RR <10 or >29 breaths/min ■ Resp distress of need for ventilation ■ Room air SpO_2 <90%	■ SBP <70 mm Hg + (2 × age)	■ SBP <90 mm Hg **OR** ■ HR > SBP	■ SBP <110 mm Hg **OR** ■ HR > SBP
Injury Patterns:	■ Penetrating injuries to head, neck, torso, proximal extremities ■ Skull deformity or suspected skull fractures ■ Suspected spinal injury w/ new motor/sensory loss ■ Chest wall unstable, deformed, or flailed ■ Suspected pelvic fractures ■ Suspected fracture on 2 or more proximal long bones ■ Crushed, degloved, mangled, or pulseless extremity ■ Amputation proximal to wrist or ankle ■ Active bleeding requiring TQ or wound pack with continuous pressure			

Patients meeting any of the above HIGH-RISK criteria should be transported to the highest-level trauma center available.

Trauma

Moderate Risk for Serious Injury

EMS Judgment:	Consider risk factors, such as:

- Low-level falls in young children (≤5 yo) or older adults (≥65 yo) with significant head impact
- Anticoagulant use
- Suspicion of child abuse
- Special, high-resource healthcare needs
- Pregnancy >20 weeks
- Burns accompanying trauma

NOTE: Children should preferentially go to pediatric-capable centers.

If concerned, take the patient to a trauma center!

Mechanism of Injury:

- High-risk auto crash
    - Partial/complete ejection
    - Significant intrusion (includes roof)
        - >12 inches occupant seat **OR**
        - >18 inches any site **OR**
        - Need for extrication
    - Death in passenger compartment
    - Child (age 0–9 yrs) unrestrained or in unsecured car seat
    - Vehicle telemetry data consistent with severe injury
- Rider separated from transport vehicle with significant impact (ATV, motorcycle, horse, etc.)
- Pedestrian/cyclist thrown, run over, or w/ significant impact
- Fall from height >10 feet (all ages)

Patients meeting any of the above MODERATE-RISK criteria WHO DO NOT MEET HIGH-RISK CRITERIA should be transported to a trauma center (need not be the highest-level trauma center).

■ Abbreviations Used in This Section

Hx—History, Signs and Symptoms
Key Symptoms and Findings (green text)
➕ — Prehospital Treatment (blue text with orange background)
Cautions—Contraindications or precautions (red text)

■ Abdominal Trauma

Hx—MOI, associated trauma, penetrating vs. blunt injury? Suspect internal hemorrhage. **Guarding**, **distension**, **rigidity**, **hypotension**, **pallor**, **bruising**?
RUQ: Liver, gall bladder, duodenum, head of pancreas, right kidney (posteriorly), ascending colon, transverse colon
LUQ: Stomach, tail of pancreas, liver, left kidney (posteriorly), spleen, transverse colon, descending colon
LLQ: Small intestine, descending colon, left ovary, fallopian tube
RLQ: Appendix, cecum, right ovary, fallopian tube, small intestine
Midline: Great vessels (aorta, vena cava), bladder, uterus
Back: Kidneys, spleen on left side
➕ —Vitals, O_2, IV, treat for shock, transport.

■ Amputation

Hx—**Time of amputation**, MOI. Vitals, hemorrhage?

⊕ —Control bleeding. Cover stump with sterile dressing, saturate with sterile saline, cover with DSD, elevate. Place severed part in plastic bag, **keep severed part dry**, place bag in ice water. If partial amputation: cover with sterile dressing, splint in anatomical position, saturate with saline, cover with DSD. O₂, *large-bore IV, titrate to vitals, ECG.*

Cautions—Time is of the essence. Transport patient and severed part to trauma center. Document PSM with times. Activate trauma team if amputation above wrist or ankle.

■ Burns

American Burn Association (ABA) Classification

Major:

- 25% TBSA or more
- 20% TBSA in children < 10 yo or adults > 40 yo
- 10% TBSA or greater full-thickness burns
- All burns involving eyes, ears, face, hands, feet, or perineum likely to cause cosmetic or functional impairment
- All high-voltage electrical burns
- Burns complicated by inhalation or major trauma
- All poor risk burn injury patients

Major burns and any burned fire fighter should be treated in a burn center.

Burn Chart

NOTE: Count only partial- or full-thickness burns.

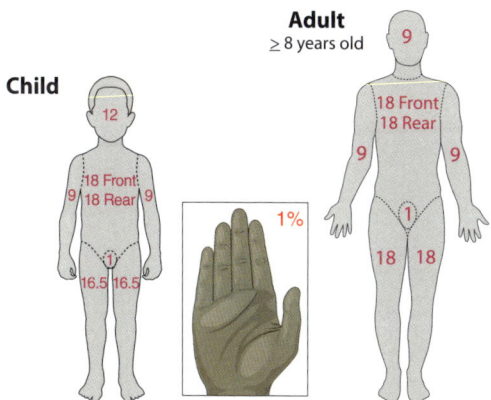

Child

Adult
≥ 8 years old

Prehospital IV Fluid Resuscitation

- < 60 min. from ED, no fluid needed
- > 60 min. transport, Lactated Ringer's:
  - ≥ 14 yo: – 500 mL/hour
  - 6–13 yo: – 250 mL/hour
  - ≤ 5 yo: – 125 mL/hour

■ Chest Trauma

NOTE: Suspect cardiac, pulmonary, or great vessel trauma.

Hx—MOI: estimate forces involved. Lung disease? **Respiratory distress**? Pain? **Use of accessory muscles**? Level of consciousness, color? GCS? Is patient anxious? **Tracheal shift**? Symmetrical chest expansion? JVD? Lung sounds? **Hemoptysis**? **Sub-Q emphysema and/or crepitus**?

Life-threatening chest injuries:
■ Flail segment   ■ Open chest wounds   ■ Tension pneumothorax

✚ —Secure airway, high-flow O_2.

✚ —**Open chest wound:** Cover with occlusive dressing. Look for exit wounds.

✚ —**Tension pneumothorax:** High-flow O_2 and rapid transport.

✚ —**Impaled objects:** Stabilize in place. Do not delay transport if patient is unstable. *Consider IV fluids for shock (two large-bore IVs), monitor ECG, vitals. Spinal immobilization, if indicated.*

Cautions—Consider other causes for respiratory distress.

■ Fractures and Dislocations

Hx —MOI. Localized pain, point tenderness, guarding, swelling, **deformity**, **angulation**, discoloration, **crepitus**, limited range of motion? Lacerations, exposed bone fragments? Distal pulses, sensation, and capillary refill?

✚ —**ABCs**, **control bleeding**, **immobilize spine as indicated by pain or MOI.** Check for additional injuries. Treat those with higher priority immediately. *Consider large-bore IV—treat shock as indicated.* Apply dressings to open wounds and splint fractures (obtain PSM before and after splinting). Elevate simple extremity fractures. Apply cold pack as needed. Monitor PSM while en route. Apply pulse oximeter to affected extremity.

Cautions—Activate trauma team for ≥ 2 proximal long bone fractures. Extremity fractures are lower priority when treating the multisystem trauma patient.

Head Trauma

Hx—MOI, estimate forces involved. Any changes in LOC? Amnesia? Was seat belt, helmet worn? Respiratory rate, pattern, quality; chest or trunk injuries? Vitals, pupils, neuro deficits? Posturing? Reflexes? Blood or CSF from ears, nose? Scalp, skull depression, associated facial trauma?

✚—Secure airway while providing C-spine immobilization if appropriate. Control bleeding with direct pressure. Do not stop bleeding from nose, ears if CSF leak is suspected. Give O_2, *start large-bore IV (TKO unless patient is in shock)*. Monitor vitals and neuro status. ECG, pulse oximetry; *manage airway if GCS ≤ 8*.

Cautions—Assess and document LOC changes. Be alert for airway problems and seizures. Restlessness and/or agitation can be due to hypoxia or hypoglycemia. Check blood glucose.

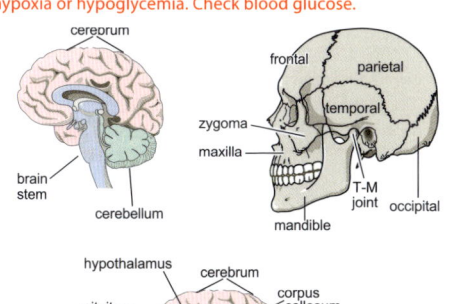

cerebrum

brain stem

cerebellum

frontal

parietal

zygoma

maxilla

temporal

T-M joint

occipital

mandible

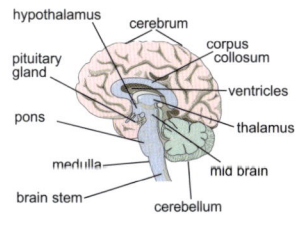

hypothalamus

cerebrum

corpus collosum

pituitary gland

ventricles

pons

thalamus

medulla

mid brain

brain stem

cerebellum

Major Bones of the Skeleton

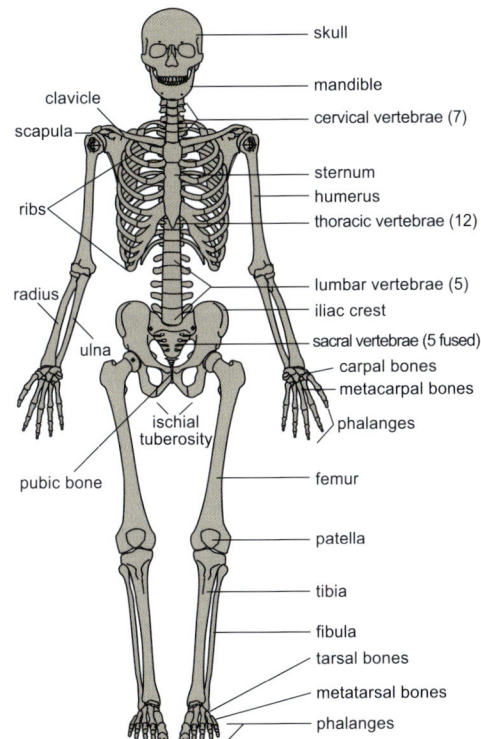

- skull
- mandible
- cervical vertebrae (7)
- clavicle
- scapula
- sternum
- humerus
- ribs
- thoracic vertebrae (12)
- radius
- lumbar vertebrae (5)
- iliac crest
- ulna
- sacral vertebrae (5 fused)
- carpal bones
- metacarpal bones
- phalanges
- ischial tuberosity
- pubic bone
- femur
- patella
- tibia
- fibula
- tarsal bones
- metatarsal bones
- phalanges

■ Spinal Injury

Hx—MOI, helmet worn? Altered mental status? Is there paralysis, weakness, numbness, tingling? Spinal pain with or without movement, point tenderness, deformity?

✚—Keep airway open. Consider nasopharyngeal airway. Immobilize per local protocol. Give O₂, if indicated. Start large-bore IV. Vitals. **Place patient in trauma system.**

■ Spinal Innervation

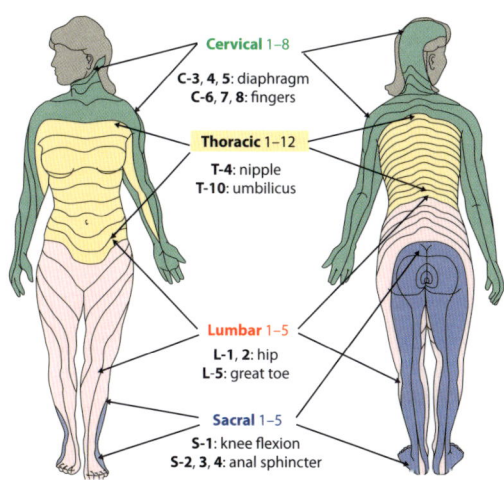

Cervical 1–8
C-3, 4, 5: diaphragm
C-6, 7, 8: fingers

Thoracic 1–12
T-4: nipple
T-10: umbilicus

Lumbar 1–5
L-1, 2: hip
L-5: great toe

Sacral 1–5
S-1: knee flexion
S-2, 3, 4: anal sphincter

■ Multiple Patients

1. **Strategically park vehicle and stay in one place.**
2. **Establish Command**, and identify yourself as Command to dispatch (use a calm, clear voice).
3. **Size up the scene** and advise dispatch of:
   - ■ Exact location and type of incident
   - ■ Any hazardous conditions
   - ■ The location of the command post
   - ■ The best routes of access to the scene
   - ■ Estimated number and severity of patients
4. **Designate an EMT to perform rapid triage.**
   Tag and number multiple patients ("**Immediate**," "**Urgent**," "**Delayed**").
5. **Order resources** (fire, police, ambulances, HazMat, extrication, air units, tow vehicles, buses, etc).
6. **Set up staging areas** (clearly state the location of staging/assembly areas, and think of access and egress).
7. **Coordinate access** of incoming units to the scene.
8. **Assign patients to incoming medical units.**
9. **Maintain communications** with OLMC.
10. **Keep patient log** indicating patient number, name, severity, treating and transporting units, medical interventions, and destination hospitals.

Crime Scene

Medical Response

CAUTION: Consider the safety of your crew first!

1. **Consider staging out of sight until scene is secure**.
2. Make a mental note of physical and weather conditions.
3. **Do not park your vehicle over visible tire tracks**.
4. Limit the number of personnel allowed on scene.

Access and Treatment

1. **Consult with police regarding best access**.
2. **To avoid destroying evidence, select a single route to and from the victim**.
3. **When moving the victim, note**:
   - Location of furniture prior to moving
   - Position of victim prior to moving
   - Status of clothing
   - Location of any weapons or other articles
   - Name of personnel who moved items
4. **Consult with police regarding whether to pick up medical debris left over from treatment**.
5. **Be conscious of any statements made**.
6. **Do NOT cut through any holes in patient's clothing**.
7. **Place victim on a clean sheet for transport. After transport, obtain the sheet, fold it onto itself, and give to the police**.
8. **Write a detailed report regarding your crew's actions**.

Scene Safety

CAUTION: Wait until police secure the scene before entering any scene of domestic violence, assault, shooting, or stabbing.

- As you approach, scan the area for hazards, such as hostile persons, dogs, uncontrolled traffic, spilled chemicals, gas, oil, or downed power lines.
- Keep your exit routes open.
- **Any weapons present at the scene should be secured**.
- **Wear protective gear. Call for more resources if needed**.

Emergency Medications

NOTE: This section is not a complete or comprehensive list of all indications, contraindications, and side effects. For complete information, please consult drug product inserts or an appropriate medical resource.

◼ Abbreviations Used in This Section

Drug Type—for medications (white/italic text)
RX—Primary indications (black text)
Contra—Primary contraindications (red text)
Dosages—(blue/bold text)
SE—Common side effects (green text)
Peds—Pediatric doses (black italic text)

◼ Emergency Medications

Activated Charcoal • *Adsorbent*

RX—Poisoning/overdose: 1 g/kg PO or by NG tube, max 100 g.
Mix with water to make a slurry.
Contra—Contact Poison Control Center for more advice.
SE—Constipation, N/V.

Albuterol 0.083% (Ventolin®) • *Bronchodilator*

RX—Bronchospasm 2° COPD, asthma: 2.5 mg/3 mL = one "fish" in nebulizer.
Contra—Tachydysrhythmias.
SE—Tachydysrhythmias, anxiety, N/V, skeletal muscle tremors.
Peds—< 10 yo: 2.5 mg (one 3-mL "fish"); ≥ 10 yo: 2.5–5 mg (one to two 3-mL "fish").
NOTE: Oxygen flow should be set at a minimum of 8 L/min. COPD patients should be monitored carefully for CO_2 retention.

Albuterol/ipratropium (Duoneb(R)) • *Bronchodilator*

RX—Bronchospasm 2° COPD, asthma: 2.5 mg albuterol + 0.5 mg ipratroplum/3 mL = one "fish" in nebulizer. May repeat.
Contra—Tachydysrhythmias.
SE—Tachydysrhythmias, anxiety, N/V.
Peds—*< 10 yo: (one 3-mL "fish"); ≥ 10 yo: (one to two 3-mL "fish").*

Aspirin (ASA) • *Antiplatelet*

RX—Acute myocardial infarction: 162–325 mg PO (2–4 chewable children's aspirin tablets).
Contra—Allergy. Use caution with asthma, ulcers, GI bleeding, other bleeding disorders, renal failure, vitamin K deficiency.
SE—GI bleeding; may exacerbate bleeding disorders.

Dextrose 10%/50% • *Nutrient*

RX—Coma, hypoglycemia (altered mental status): 125–250 mL D10% **OR** 25–50 mL D50%, slow IV/IO. Can give orally.
SE—Anxiety, tremor, headache, tachycardia, palpitations, PVCs, angina, hypertension. Extravasation of dextrose 50% will cause necrosis of tissue. Hyperglycemia may complicate or worsen many of medical/traumatic conditions (i.e. myocardial infarction, stroke). Dextrose 50%/10% should be given whenever hypoglycemia is documented by glucometry.
D10% is preferred for IV/IO routes.
Contra—Intracerebral bleeding, hemorrhagic CVA.
Peds—*Hypoglycemia (altered mental status): 5 mL/kg D10%, max 250 mL D10% slow IV/IO. May repeat once. Can give orally.*

Epinephrine (Adrenalin®) • *Sympathomimetic*

RX—Allergic reaction: 0.3–0.5 mg (0.3–0.5 mL 1 mg/mL or 1:1,000) IM/IV/IO may repeat once in 5–15 min **OR** 1 mg/10 mL (1:10,000) 0.1 mg bolus IV/IO every 3–5 min; titrate to effect, **max total dose** 0.5 mg
RX—Asthma: 0.3–0.5 mg (0.3–0.5 mL 1 mg/mL or 1:1,000) **IM**.

RX—Ventricular fibrillation, asystole, PEA: 1 mg IV/IO 1 mg (10 mL of 0.1 mg/mL 1:10,000) **repeat q 3–5 min.**
Contra—Tachydysrhythmias, severe coronary artery disease.
SE—Tachydysrhythmias, VT, VF angina, HTN, N/V, anxiety.
Peds—**RX—Allergic reaction:** 0.01 mg/kg of 1 mg/mL (1:1,000) IM; may repeat x1 in 5–15 min, **max total dose** 0.5 mg.
OR
1 mg/10 mL (1:10,000) 0.01 mg/kg (**max** 0.1 mg) IV bolus every 3–5 min titrated to effect, **max total dose** 0.5 mg
RX—Asthma: 0.01 mg/kg of 1 mg/mL (1:1,000) IM, **max total dose** 0.5 mg.

Epinephrine (EpiPen®) • *Bronchodilator/Vasoconstrictor*

RX—Allergic reaction: 0.3 mg IM.
Contra—Tachydysrhythmias, severe coronary artery disease.
SE—Tachydysrhythmias, VT, VF angina, HTN, N/V, anxiety.
Peds—*EpiPen Jr®: 0.15 mg IM.*

Glucagon • ↑ *Blood Glucose*

RX—Hypoglycemia: **1 mg IM**. Give carbohydrate (prompt meal, orange juice, D50%, etc) as soon as the patient is alert and can eat.
Peds—*0.02 mg/kg IM*, ***max total dose*** *1.0 mg.*

Oral Glucose (Glutose®) • *Nutrient*

RX—Hypoglycemia: **15–25 g** (**one tube**) **PO**.
SE—Patient may aspirate if no gag reflex present.
Contra—Patient must be awake enough to swallow. Protect patient's airway.

◼ IV Solutions

5% Dextrose in Water (D₅W) • *Hypotonic Dextrose Solution*

RX—IV access and diluent for medications: **microdrip (60 gtt/mL) set at TKO.**
Contra—Hypovolemia. Do not use with phenytoin (Dilantin).
SE—Rare in therapeutic dosages.

Lactated Ringer's • *Isotonic Crystalloid Solution*

RX—Hypovolemic shock, burns: **run rapidly**. In other cases: **administer at moderate rate, 100 cc/hour**.
Contra—HF or renal failure.
SE—Rare in therapeutic dosages

0.9% Sodium Chloride (Normal Saline) • *Isotonic Crystalloid Solution*

RX—Hypovolemia, diabetic ketoacidosis, freshwater drowning, heatstroke: **run rapidly**. In other cases: **administer at moderate rate, 100 cc/hour.**
Contra—HF, circulatory overload.
SE—Rare in therapeutic dosages.

Naloxone • *Opioid Antagonist*

RX—**Opiate overdose; coma:** If no IV present: **2–4 mg IM/intranasal** is sufficient to reverse opioid intoxication.
If IV present: **0.5 mg IV/IO may be repeated q 2 min up to 2 mg.** In some cases, larger doses may be required (for methadone or designer drugs). In these cases, administer additional doses of naloxone (**2 mg IM/intranasal or IV/IO q 3–5 minutes up to max total dose of 8 mg**). If no reaction, consider other causes.
Contra—Do not use on a newborn if the mother is addicted to narcotics; may cause withdrawal.
SE—Withdrawal symptoms in the addicted patient, APE, N/V, ↓BP, HTN, seizure.
Peds—< 20 kg: 0.1 mg/kg IV/IO/IM, no more than 2 mg/dose. Do not use in neonates.

Nitroglycerin • *Vasodilator*

RX—**Acute angina**, **hypertension**, **HF with APE**.
Contra—Hypotension; hypovolemia; intracranial bleeding; recent use of Viagra®, Cialis®, or Levitra®.
SE Headache, hypotension, syncope, tachycardia, flushing.
Nitro tablets (Nitrostat®): 0.4 mg SL, may repeat q 5 minutes if SBP > 100.

Nitroglycerin spray (Nitrolingual®): 1–2 sprays (0.4–0.8 mg) **under the tongue.**

Nitroglycerin paste (Nitro-Bid®): 1–2 cm of paste (6–12 mg) **topically.**

Nitrous Oxide (Nitronox®) • *Analgesic*

RX—Analgesia/sedation: Give mask to patient and allow to self-administer.

Contra—↓LOC, cyanosis, acute abdomen, shock, ↓BP, pneumothorax, chest trauma, patients who need > 50% O_2.

SE—Drowsiness, euphoria, apnea, N/V.

NOTE: Ventilate patient area during use.

Oxygen

	Liters/Minute	O_2 Delivered
Nasal Cannula	1	24%
	2	28%
	4	36%
	6	44%
Face Mask	6	50%–60%
NRB Mask	10	80%
	15	90%
Pocket Mask	Mouth-to-mask	17%
	10	50%
	15	80%
	30	100%
Bag-Valve-Mask (with reservoir)	Room air	21%
	10	90%
	15	95%
Positive Pressure	100	100%

Contra—COPD patients may become apneic with high-flow O_2.

Pulse Oximetry

Ranges	Prehospital Treatment
Normal: 95%–99%	
Mild hypoxia: 91%–94%	Give oxygen
Moderate hypoxia: 86%–90%	Give high-flow oxygen
Severe hypoxia: ≤ 85%	100% oxygen, ventilate

Falsely low SpO$_2$ readings may be caused by:
- Cold extremities
- Excessive movement
- Low perfusion

Falsely high SpO$_2$ readings may be caused by:
- Anemia
- Carbon monoxide poisoning

If in doubt, give oxygen in spite of a normal SpO$_2$.

O$_2$ Tank Capacities

Tank	Capacity	@15 Lpm	10 Lpm	6 Lpm	2 Lpm
C	240 L	16 minutes	24 minutes	40 minutes	2 hours
D	360 L	24 minutes	36 minutes	1 hour	3 hours
E	625 L	41 minutes	1:02 hours	1:44 hours	5:12 hours
M	3000 L	3:20 hours	5:00 hours	8:20 hours	25 hours
G	5300 L	5:53 hours	8:50 hours	14:43 hours	44:10 hours
H	6900 L	7:40 hours	11:30 hours	19:10 hours	57:30 hours

Medications

IV Fluid Rates in Drops/Minute

Drip Set	10	12	15	20	60*
30 mL/hour	5	6	8	10	30
60 mL/hour	10	12	15	20	60
100 mL/hour	17	20	25	33	100
200 mL/hour	33	40	50	67	200
300 mL/hour	50	60	75	100	300
400 mL/hour	67	80	100	133	400
500 mL/hour	83	100	125	167	500
1000 mL/hour	167	200	250	333	1000

*Standard "microdrip" IV tubing has 60 gtt/mL.
A normal TKO or KVO rate is 30–50 mL/hour.
Note that with a microdrip IV set, mL/hour = drops/minute.

Prescription Drugs

NOTE: All caps is brand names and title caps is generic.

A

ABILIFY (aripiprazole): antipsychotic; Rx: schizophrenia

Abrocitinib (CIBINQO): dermatologic; Rx: atopic dermatitis in adults

Acarbose: oral hypoglycemic; Rx: diabetes

ACCOLATE (zafirlukast): bronchospasm inhibitor; Rx: asthma

ACCUPRIL (quinapril): ACE inhibitor; Rx: HTN, HF

ACCURETIC (quinapril/HCTZ): ACE inhibitor/diuretic; Rx: HTN

Acebutolol: β-blocker; Rx: HTN, angina, dysrhythmias

Acetaminophen (TYLENOL): non-narcotic analgesic

Acetazolamide: diuretic/anticonvulsant; Rx: glaucoma, edema in HF, epilepsy, mountain sickness

ACIPHEX (rabeprazole): inhibits gastric acid secretion; Rx: ulcers, GERD, Zollinger-Ellison syndrome

ACLOVATE (alclometasone): topical corticosteroid; Rx: rashes, psoriasis

ACTIQ (fentanyl): oral transmucosal narcotic analgesic; Rx: chronic cancer pain

ACTONEL (risedronate): reduces bone loss; Rx: osteoporosis, Paget's disease

ACTOS (pioglitazone): oral hypoglycemic; Rx: diabetes

Acyclovir (ZOVIRAX): antiviral; Rx: herpes, shingles, chicken pox

ADDERALL (amphetamine/dextroamphetamine): CNS stimulant; Rx: ADHD, narcolepsy

ADLYXIN (lixisenatide): antidiabetic; Rx: diabetes

ADRENALIN (epinephrine): bronchodilator, vasopressor; Rx: asthma, life threatening allergic reactions, anaphylaxis

ADVAIR DISKUS (fluticasone/salmeterol): inhaled steroid/β-2 bronchodilator; Rx: asthma, COPD

AEMCOLO (rifamycin): antibiotic; Rx: travelers' diarrhea

AIMOVIG (erenumab-aooe): antimigraine; Rx: migraine prevention

AJOVY (fremanezumab-vfrm): antimigraine; Rx: migraine prevention

Albuterol HFA (PROVENTIL inhalation): β-2 agonist bronchodilator; Rx: asthma, COPD

ALDACTAZIDE (spironolactone/HCTZ): diuretics; Rx: HTN, fluid retention

ALDACTONE (spironolactone): potassium-sparing diuretic; Rx: HF, ESLD, HTN

Alendronate (FOSOMAX): reduces bone loss; Rx: osteoporosis, Paget's disease

Alirocumab (PRALUENT): monoclonal antibody; Rx: hypercholesterolemia

ALLEGRA (fexofenadine): antihistamine; Rx: allergies

Allopurinol (ZYLOPRIM): xanthine oxidase inhibitor; Rx: gout

Alosetron (LOTRONEX): antidiarrheal; Rx: irritable bowel

Alprazolam (XANAX): benzodiazepine; Rx: anxiety disorders, panic attacks

ALTACE (ramipril): ACE inhibitor; Rx: HTN, HF post MI

ALTOPREV (lovastatin): statin; Rx: hypercholesterolemia, HF

Amantadine: anticholinergic, antiviral, antiparkinsonian; Rx: influenza A, Parkinson's disease

AMARYL (glimepiride): oral hypoglycemic; Rx: diabetes mellitus

AMBIEN (zolpidem): sedative; Rx: insomnia

AMERGE (naratriptan): selective serotonin receptor agonist; Rx: acute migraine H/A

Amiloride: diuretic; Rx: HTN, fluid retention

Amiloride/HCTZ: diuretics; Rx: HTN, fluid retention

Aminophylline: bronchodilator; Rx: COPD, asthma, bronchitis

Amiodarone (PACERONE): antiarrhythmic; Rx: dysrhythmias

AMITIZA (lubiprostone): intestinal stimulant; Rx: chronic idiopathic constipation

Amitriptyline (ELAVIL): tricyclic antidepressant; Rx: depression, neuropathic pain

Amlodipine/benazepril (LOTREL): calcium channel blocker; Rx: HTN, angina

Amoxapine (ASENDIN): tricyclic antidepressant

Amoxicillin: penicillin class antibiotic

Amoxicillin/clavulanate: penicillin class antibiotic

Amphetamine (ADDERALL): stimulant; Rx: ADHD

Amphotericin B: antifungal agent; Rx: fungal infections

Ampicillin: penicillin class antibiotic

ANAFRANIL (clomipramine): tricyclic antidepressant; Rx: obsessive-compulsive disorder

ANAPROX DS (naproxen): NSAID analgesic; Rx: arthritis, pain

ANTIVERT/BONINE (meclizine): antiemetic, antihistamine; Rx: motion sickness

ARANESP (darbepoetin alfa): erythropoiesis stimulating agent; Rx: anemia

ARAVA (leflunomide): immunomodulator agent; Rx: rheumatoid arthritis

ARICEPT (donepezil): cholinergic enhancer; Rx: dementia associated with Alzheimer's

Aripiprazole lauroxil (ARISTADA): antipsychotic; Rx: schizophrenia

ARISTADA (aripiprazole lauroxil): antipsychotic; Rx: schizophrenia

ARIXTRA (fondaparinux): anticoagulant; Rx: treatment and prophylaxis for DVT/PE

ARMOUR THYROID: thyroid desiccated; Rx: hypothyroidism

ARTHROTEC (diclofenac/misoprostol): NSAID analgesic, antiulcer; Rx: arthritis

Aspirin (salicylate, acetylsalicylic acid, ASA): NSAID analgesic; Rx: pain

ATACAND (candesartan/cilexetil): angiotensin receptor blockers; Rx: HTN, HF

Atenolol (TENORMIN): β-blocker; Rx: HTN, angina, AMI

Atenolol/chlorthalidone (TENORETIC 100, TENORETIC 50): β-blocker/diuretic; Rx: HTN

ATIVAN (lorazepam): benzodiazepine hypnotic; Rx: anxiety

Atovaquone (MEPRON): antiparasitic; Rx: prophylaxis and treatment for *Pneumocystis* pneumonia (PCP)

ATROVENT HFA (ipratropium inhalation): inhaled anticholinergic bronchodilator; Rx: COPD, asthma exacerbation

AVALIDE (irbesartan/hydrochlorothiazide): angiotensin receptor blocker/diuretic; Rx: HTN

AVANDAMET (rosiglitazone/metformin): oral hypoglycemic combination; Rx: diabetes

AVAPRO (irbesartan): angiotensin receptor blocker; Rx: HTN, diabetic nephropathy

AVODART (dutasteride): androgen inhibitor; Rx: benign prostatic hypertrophy

AVONEX (interferon-β-1a): immunonodulator; Rx: multiple sclerosis

AYGESTIN (norethindrone acetate): hormone; Rx: amenorrhea, endometriosis

AZACTAM (aztreonam): monobactam antibiotic; Rx: bacterial infections, pneumonia, UTI

Azathioprine (IMURAN): immunosuppressant; Rx: organ transplants, lupus, rheumatoid arthritis

Azelastine (OPTIVAR): antihistamine; Rx: hay fever, allergies

AZILECT (rasagiline): MAO-B inhibitor, slows metabolism of dopamine; Rx: Parkinson's disease

Azithromycin (ZITHROMAX): macrolide antibiotic; Rx: bacterial infection

AZOPT (brinzolamide OPTH): carbonic anhydrase inhibitor; Rx: glaucoma, ocular hypertension

Aztreonam (AZACTAM): monobactam antibiotic; Rx: bacterial infections

AZULFIDINE-EN-Tabs (sulfasalazine): anti-inflammatory; Rx: ulcerative colitis, arthritis

B

B & O SUP (belladonna, opium): antispasmodic/analgesic; Rx: ureteral spasm pain

Bacitracin: topical antibiotic; Rx: prevention/treatment of superficial infections

Bacitracin/neomycin/polymyxin/B/hydrocortisone (CORTISPORIN): topical antibiotics/steroid; Rx: skin infection/inflammation

Bacitracin/polymyxin (POLYSPORIN): topical antibiotic

Baclofen: muscle relaxant; Rx: spasm in MS, spinal cord disease

BACTRIM (trimethoprim/sulfamethoxazole): sulfa antibacterial compound; Rx: bacterial infections

Baloxavir marboxil (XOFLUZA): antiviral; Rx: influenza

Balsalazide (COLAZAL): anti-inflammatory; Rx: ulcerative colitis

Baricitnib (OLUMIANT): antirheumatic; Rx: rheumatoid arthritis

Beclomethasone: inhaled corticosteroid; Rx: asthma

BECONASE AQ (beclomethasone nasal): nasal steroid; Rx: allergies

Belladonna alkaloids w/phenobarbital (DONNATAL): antispasmodic; Rx: irritable bowel, ulcers in the intestines

Benazepril (LOTENSIN): ACE inhibitor; Rx: HTN

Benazepril/HCTZ (LOTENSIN HCT): ACE inhibitor/diuretic; Rx: HTN

BENICAR (olmesartan): angiotensin II receptor antagonist; Rx: HTN

BENTYL (dicyclomine): anticholinergic; Rx: irritable bowel

Benzonatate: antitussive; Rx: cough

Benzphetamine: amphetamine; Rx: obesity

Benztropine: anticholinergic; Rx: Parkinson's disease, extrapyramidal disorders

BETAGAN (levobunolol opth): β-blocker, lowers intraocular pressure; Rx: glaucoma

Betamethasone (CELESTONE, SOLUSPAN): corticosteroid anti-inflammatory

BETAPACE (sotalol): antiarrhythmic; Rx: dysrhythmias, β-blocker

BETASERON (interferon-β-1b): immunomodulator; Rx: multiple sclerosis

Betaxolol: β-blocker; Rx: HTN

Bethanechol: urinary cholinergic; Rx: urinary retention

BETOPTIC/BETOPTIC S (betaxolol ophthalmic): β-blocker; Rx: glaucoma

Brexanolone (ZULRESSO): antidepressant; Rx: postpartum depression

Brexpiprazole (REXULTI): antipsychotic; Rx: schizophrenia

BICILLIN (penicillin): penicillin antibiotic; Rx: bacterial infections

BIDIL (hydralazine/isosorbide dinitrate): vasodilators; Rx: heart failure

Bisacodyl (DULCOLAX): laxative; Rx: constipation

Bismuth subsalicylate (PEPTO-BISMOL): gastrointestinal; Rx: indigestion, diarrhea

Bisoprolol: β-blocker; Rx: HTN

Bisoprolol/HCTZ: β-blocker/diuretic; Rx: HTN

BONIVA (ibandronate): osteoclast inhibitor; Rx: osteoporosis

Brimonidine ophthalmic (ALPHAGAN P): α-adrenergic agonist; Rx: glaucoma, ocular hypertension

Brinzolamide ophthalmic (AZOPT): α-adrenergic agonist; Rx: glaucoma, ocular hypertension

Bromocriptine (PARLODEL): dopamine agonist; Rx: Parkinson's disease, hyperprolactinemia, acromegaly

Brompheniramine/phenylephrine: antihistamine, decongestant, α-1 agonist; Rx: allergies

Budesonide (ENTOCORT EC): nasal, inhaled corticosteroid; Rx: allergic rhinitis, asthma

Bumetanide: diuretic; Rx: edema, HF

BUPAP (butalbital, acetaminophen): sedative analgesic, antipyretic; Rx: tension headache

Buprenorphine: opioid partial agonist antagonist; Rx: opioid dependence

Bupropion (WELLBUTRIN SR): antidepressant; Rx: depression, smoking cessation, norepinephrine-dopamine reuptake inhibitor

Buspirone: antianxiety agent; Rx: anxiety disorders, serotonin-dopamine modulator

Busulfan (MYLERAN): anticancer agent; Rx: chronic myelogenous leukemia, immunosuppresive oncologic agent

Butalbital/acetaminophen/caffeine (FIORICET/ESGIC): sedative analgesic; Rx: tension headaches

Butalbital/aspirin/caffeine (FIORINAL): sedative analgesic; Rx: tension headache

Butorphanol: opioid analgesic; Rx: pain

BYETTA (exenatide): enhances insulin secretion; Rx: type 2 diabetes

CADUET (amlodipine/atorvastatin): calcium blocker/lipid-lowering agent; Rx: HTN, high cholesterol

CAFERGOT (ergotamine/caffeine): vasoconstrictor; Rx: migraine/tension H/A

CALAN, CALAN SR (verapamil): calcium channel blocker; Rx: angina, hypertension, prophylaxis headache, dysrhythmias

CALCIFEROL (ergocalciferol, vitamin D2): vitamin D; Rx: hypocalcemia, hypoparathyroidism, rickets, osteodystrophy

Calcipotriene: vitamin D agonist; Rx: psoriasis

Calcitonin-salmon (MIACALCIN): bone resorption inhibitor hormone; Rx: hypercalcemia, Paget's disease, osteoporosis

Calcitriol (ROCALTROL): vitamin D supplement; Rx: hypocalcemia in renal disease, hypoparathyroidism, bone disease

Candesartan/cilexetil (ATACAND): ACE inhibitor, angiotensin receptor blocker; Rx: HTN, HF

CAPLYTA (lumateperone tosylate): antipsychotic; Rx: schizophremia

Capsaicin topical (QUZENTA): topical analgesic; Rx: muscle/joint pain including arthritis

Captopril: ACE inhibitor; Rx: HTN, HF, diabetic nephropathy

CARAFATE (sucralfate): gastrointestinal agent; Rx: duodenal ulcer

Carbamazepine (CARBATROL, TEGRETOL): anticonvulsant; Rx: Sz, trigeminal neuralgia, bipolar disorder

CARBATROL (carbamazepine): anticonvulsant; Rx: seizures, trigeminal neuralgia, bipolar disorder

Carbidopa/levodopa (SINEMET, RYTARY): dopamine precursor; Rx: Parkinson's disease

CARDIZEM (diltiazem): calcium channel blocker; Rx: angina, HTN

CARDURA (doxazosin): α-blocker; Rx: HTN, benign prostatic hypertrophy

Cariprazine (VRAYLAR): antipsychotic; Rx: schizophrenia and bipolar disorder

Carisoprodol (SOMA): muscle relaxant; Rx: musculoskeletal pain

Carvedilol (COREG): β-adrenergic blocker; Rx: angina, heart failure, HTN

CASODEX (bicalutamide): antiandrogen; Rx: prostate cancer

CATAPRES TTS (clonidine transdermal): centrally acting α agonist; Rx: HTN

Cefaclor: cephalosporin antibiotic; Rx: bacterial infections

Cefadroxil: cephalosporin antibiotic; Rx: bacterial infections

Cefazolin: cephalosporin antibiotic; Rx: bacterial infections

Cefdinir: cephalosporin antibiotic; Rx: bacterial infections

Cefepime: cephalosporin antibiotic; Rx: bacterial infections

Cefixime (SUPRAX): cephalosporin antibiotic; Rx: bacterial infections

Cefotetan: cephalosporin antibiotic; Rx: bacterial infections

Cefoxitin: cephalosporin antibiotic; Rx: bacterial infections

Cefpodoxime: cephalosporin antibiotic; Rx: bacterial infections

Cefprozil: cephalosporin antibiotic; Rx: bacterial infections

Ceftazidime (FORTAZ): cephalosporin antibiotic; Rx: bacterial infections

Ceftizoxime: cephalosporin antibiotic; Rx: bacterial infections

Cefuroxime: cephalosporin antibiotic; Rx: bacterial infections

CELEBREX (celecoxib): NSAID; Rx: arthritis, acute pain

CELEXA (citalopram): SSRI; Rx: depression

CEREBYX (fosphenytoin): anticonvulsant; Rx: epilepsy

Cetirizine (ZYRTEC): antihistamine; Rx: allergic rhinitis, urticaria

Chlordiazepoxide: benzodiazepine; Rx: anxiety, agitation from alcohol withdrawal

Chloroquine phosphate: antimalarial, amebicidal agent; Rx: malaria

Chlorothiazide (DIURIL): diuretic; Rx: fluid retention in HF, renal failure, HTN

Chlorpheniramine (CHLOR-TRIMETON): antihistamine; Rx: colds, allergies

Chlorpromazine: antipsychotic; Rx: schizophrenia

Chlorthalidone: diuretic; Rx: fluid retention in HF, renal failure, HTN

Chlorzoxazone: skeletal muscle relaxant

Cholestyramine (QUESTRAN): bile acid sequestrant; Rx: antihyperlipidemic, pruritus/urticaria

CIALIS (tadalafil): vasodilator; Rx: male erectile dysfunction

CIBINQO (abrocitinib): dermatologic; Rx: atopic dermatitis in adults

Cidofovir: antiviral; Rx: cytomegalovirus in AIDS

Cilostazol: vasodilator, platelet inhibitor; Rx: leg cramps

Cimetidine (TAGAMET HB): H-2 blocker, inhibits gastric acid secretion; Rx: ulcers

CINQAIR (reslizumab): monoclonal antibody; Rx: severe asthma

CIPRO (ciprofloxacin): fluoroquinolone antibiotic; Rx: bacterial infections

Ciprofloxacin (CIPRO): fluoroquinolone antibiotic; Rx: bacterial infections

Citalopram (CELEXA): SSRI; Rx: depression

CLARINEX (desloratadine): antihistamine; Rx: urticaria, allergies

Clarithromycin: macrolide antibiotic; Rx: bacterial infections

CLIMARA (estradiol): transdermal estrogen; Rx: symptoms of menopause

Clindamycin (CLEOCIN): antibiotic; Rx: bacterial infections

Clobetasol: topical steroid anti-inflammatory; Rx: dermatoses

Clomipramine (ANAFRANIL): tricyclic antidepressant; Rx: obsessive compulsive disorder

Clonazepam (KLONOPIN): benzodiazepine, anticonvulsant; Rx: Sz, panic disorders

Clonidine transdermal (CATAPRES TTS): centrally acting α agonist; Rx: HTN

Clopidogrel (PLAVIX): antiplatelet; Rx: ACS, AMI, stroke

Clorazepate: benzodiazepine; Rx: anxiety/Sz

Clotrimazole (LOTRIMIN AF): antifungal; Rx: fungal infection

Clotrimazole/betamethasone: topical antifungal/corticosteroid; Rx: fungal infection

Clozapine (CLOZARIL): antipsychotic; Rx: schizophrenia

CLOZARIL (clozapine): antipsychotic; Rx: schizophrenia

Codeine: narcotic analgesic/antitussive

COGNEX (tacrine): cholinesterase inhibitor; Rx: Alzheimer's disease

COLACE (docusate): stool softener; Rx: constipation

COLAZAL (balsalazide): anti-inflammatory; Rx: ulcerative colitis

Colchicine: anti-inflammatory; Rx: gout

Colesevelam (WELCHOL): bile acid sequestrant; Rx: hyperlipidemia

COLESTID (colestipol): bile acid sequestrant; Rx: hyperlipidemia

Colestipol (COLESTID): bile acid sequestrant; Rx: hyperlipidemia

Colistimethate (COLY-MYCIN M): antibiotic; Rx: *Pseudomonas* infection

COLY-MYCIN M (colistimethane): antibiotic; Rx: *Pseudomonas* infection

COMBIPATCH (estradiol, norethindrone): estrogen; Rx: menopause symptoms

COMBIVIR (lamivudine/zidovudine): antiretroviral; Rx: HIV

COMTAN (entacapone): COMT inhibitor; Rx: Parkinson's disease

CONCERTA (methylphenidate): CNS stimulant; Rx: ADHD, narcolepsy

CONTRAVE (naltrexone/bupropion): antidepressant; Rx: weight management

COPAXONE (glatiramer): immunomodulator; Rx: MS

COREG (carvedilol): β-adrenergic blocker; Rx: HTN, HF, angina

CORGARD (nadolol): β-blocker; Rx: HTN, angina

CORTIFOAM (hydrocortisone): steroid anti-inflammatory; Rx: proctitis, various skin conditions

CORTISOL (hydrocortisone): steroid anti-inflammatory; Rx: arthritis, allergies, asthma, inflammatory bowel disease

Cortisone: steroid anti-inflammatory; Rx: various skin conditions, allergies, adrenal insufficiency

CORVERT (ibutilide): antiarrhythmic; Rx: atrial fibrillation, flutter

COSOPT (timolol/dorzolamide OPTH): decreases intraocular pressure; Rx: glaucoma

COZAAR (losartan): angiotensin receptor blocker; Rx: HTN, diabetic nephropathy

CREON, CREON 5, CREON 10, CREON 20 (pancrelipase): pancreatic enzyme replacement

CRESTOR (rosuvastatin): statin; Rx: hyperlipidemia

CRIXIVAN (indinavir): protease inhibitor antiretroviral; Rx: HIV

Cyanocobalamin (vitamin B12): Rx: anemia

Cyclobenzaprine: skeletal muscle relaxant

Cyclosporine (GENGRAF, NEORAL, SANDIMMUNE): immunosuppressant agent; Rx: organ transplants

CYMBALTA (duloxetine): SNRI, SSRI; Rx: depression, diabetic neuropathy

Cyproheptadine: antihistamine; Rx: seasonal allergies

CYTOMEL (liothyronine): thyroid hormone; Rx: hypothyroidism

CYTOTEC (misoprostol): prevents gastric ulcers from NSAIDs

CYTOVENE (ganciclovir): antiviral; Rx: CMV disease (cytomegalovirus)

D

Danazol: sex hormone; Rx: endometriosis

DANTRIUM (dantrolene): skeletal muscle antispasmodic; Rx: spasm, malignant hyperthermia

Dantrolene (DANTRIUM): skeletal muscle antispasmodic; Rx: spasm, malignant hyperthermia

Dapsone: antibacterial drug; Rx: leprosy, PCP prophylaxis

DARAPRIM (pyrimethamine): antiparasitic; Rx: malaria, toxoplasmosis

DAYVIGO (lemborexant): hypnotic; Rx: insomnia

DAYPRO (oxaprozin): NSAID; Rx: arthritis

Delavirdine: antiretroviral; Rx: HIV

DEMEROL (meperidine): opioid analgesic; Rx: moderate-to-severe pain

DENAVIR (penciclovir): topical antiviral; Rx: herpes, cold sores

DEPAKOTE, DEPAKOTE ER (divalproex): anticonvulsant, antimigraine; Rx: migraine headache, absence seizures

DEPO-MEDROL (methylprednisolone): corticosteroid anti-inflammatory

Desipramine (NORPRAMIN): tricyclic antidepressant

Desonide (DESOWEN): topical corticosteroid; Rx: dermatoses

Desoximetasone (TOPICORT): topical corticosteroid; Rx: dermatoses

DESOXYN (methamphetamine): amphetamine; Rx: ADHD, obesity

DETROL (tolterodine): anticholinergic, urinary bladder antispasmodic; Rx: overactive bladder

Dexamethasone: steroid anti-inflammatory; Rx: neoplastic disorders, allergies, GI diseases, endocrine disorders

DEXEDRINE (dextroamphetamine): amphetamine; Rx: ADHD, narcolepsy

Dextroamphetamine (DEXEDRINE): amphetamine; Rx: ADHD, narcolepsy

Dextroamphetamine/amphetamine (ADDERALL): amphetamine; Rx: ADHD, narcolepsy

Dextromethorphan (DELSYM, ROBITUSSIN): non-narcotic antitussive

Diazepam (VALIUM): benzodiazepine; Rx: anxiety, Sz, panic disorder

Diclofenac: NSAID, analgesic; Rx: arthritis, inflammation

Dicloxacillin: penicillin antibiotic; Rx: bacterial infections

Dicyclomine (BENTYL): anticholinergic; Rx: irritable bowel syndrome

DIFLUCAN (fluconazole): antifungal; Rx: yeast infection

Diflunisal: NSAID analgesic; Rx: arthritis

DIGITEK (digoxin): cardiac glycoside; Rx: HF, atrial fibrillation

Digoxin (DIGITEK LANOXIN): cardiac glycoside; Rx: HF, atrial fibrillation

Dihydroergotamine (D.H.E.): ergot alkaloid, vasoconstrictor; Rx: migraine H/A

DILANTIN (phenytoin): anticonvulsant; Rx: Sz

DILAUDID (hydromorphone): opioid analgesic; Rx: moderate-to-severe pain

Diltiazem (CARDIZEM): calcium channel blocker; Rx: angina, HTN, PSVT

Dimenhydrinate (DRAMAMINE): antihistamine; Rx: motion sickness

DIOVAN (valsartan): angiotensin II receptor inhibitor; Rx: HTN, HF post MI

DIOVAN HCT (valsartan/HCTZ): angiotensin II receptor inhibitor/diuretic; Rx: HTN

DIPENTUM (olsalazine): anti-inflammatory agent; Rx: ulcerative colitis

Diphenhydramine (BENADRYL): antihistamine; Rx: allergies

Diphenoxylate/atropine (LOMOTIL): opioid congener; Rx: diarrhea

Dipyridamole: antiplatelet; Rx: lowers risk of postoperative thromboembolic complications after heart valve replacement

Disopyramide (NORPACE): antiarrhythmic; Rx: ventricular dysrhythmias

Disulfiram: alcohol-abuse deterrent; Rx: alcohol abuse

DITROPAN XL (oxybutynin): anticholinergic/antispasmodic; Rx: urinary frequency, incontinence, dysuria

DIURIL (chlorothiazide): diuretic; Rx: fluid retention in HF, renal failure, HTN

Divalproex (DEPAKOTE): anticonvulsant; Rx: seizures, bipolar disorder, migraines

Docusate (COLACE): stool softener; Rx: constipation

Dolasetron: antiemetic; Rx: nausea and vomiting

Donepezil (ARICEPT): cholinergic; Rx: dementia associated with Alzheimer's disease

DONNATAL (phenobarbital/belladonna alkaloids): barbiturate sedative/antispasmodic; Rx: irritable bowel syndrome

Doravirine (PIFELTRO): antiretroviral; Rx: HIV infection

Dornase alfa (PULMOZYME): inhaled lytic enzyme that dissolves infected lung secretions; Rx: cystic fibrosis

Dorzolamide OPTH (TRUSOPT): decreases intraocular pressure; Rx: glaucoma

Dorzolamide/timolol OPTH (COSOPT): decreases intraocular pressure; Rx: glaucoma

Doxazosin (CARDURA): α-blocker; Rx: HTN, benign prostatic hypertrophy

Doxepin: tricyclic antidepressant; Rx: depression, anxiety

DOXIL (doxorubicin): antineoplastic; Rx: AIDS-related tumors, cancer, leukemia

Doxycycline (VIBRAMYCIN): tetracycline antibiotic; Rx: bacterial infections

Doxylamine (UNISOM): antihistamine sedative; Rx: insomnia

DRAMAMINE (dimenhydrinate): antihistamine; Rx: motion sickness

Dronabinol (MARINOL): cannabinoid appetite stimulant; Rx: weight loss in cancer, AIDS

DUONEB (ipratropium/albuterol): bronchodilators; Rx: asthma, COPD

Dupilumab (DUPIXENT): monoclonal antibody; Rx: atopic dermatitis

DUPIXENT (dupilumab): monoclonal antibody; Rx: atopic dermatitis

DURAMORPH (morphine): opioid analgesic; Rx: moderate-to-severe pain

DYRENIUM (triamterene): potassium-sparing diuretic; Rx: edema in HF/ESLD/nephrotic syndrome

E

Econazole: topical antifungal; Rx: fungal infections

EDECRIN (ethacrynic acid): diuretic; Rx: HF, pulmonary edema

Edoxaban (SAVAYSA): anticoagulant; Rx: atrial fibrillation

EDLUAR (zolpidem): sedative; Rx: insomnia

E.E.S. (erythromycin): macrolide antibiotic; Rx: bacterial infection

Efavirenz (SUSTIVA): antiviral; Rx: HIV-I infection

EFFEXOR, EFFEXOR XR (venlafaxine): antidepressant; Rx: depression, anxiety, panic disorder

ELOCON (mometasone): topical corticosteroid; Rx: dermatoses

Eluxadoline (VIBERZI): GI agent; Rx: irritable bowel syndrome

EMGALITY (galcanezumab-gnlm): antimigraine; Rx: migraine prevention

EMSAM patch (selegiline): MAO inhibitor; Rx: depression

EMTRIVA (emtricitabine): antiretroviral; Rx: HIV

ENABLEX (darifenacin): anticholinergic; Rx: overactive bladder

Enalapril, enalaprilat (VASOTEC): ACE inhibitor; Rx: HTN, HF

Enalapril/HCTZ: ACE inhibitor/diuretic; Rx: HTN

ENBREL (etanercept): immunomdulator; Rx: arthritis; psoriasis

ENDOCET (oxycodone/acetaminophen): opioid analgesic; Rx: moderate-to-severe pain

Entacapone (COMTAN): COMT inhibitor; Rx: Parkinson's disease

ENTEREG (alvimopan): GI opioid antagonist; Rx: postoperative ileus

ENTOCORT EC (budesonide): corticosteroid; Rx: Crohn's disease

ENTRESTO (sacubitril/valsartan): angiotensin II blocker; Rx: heart failure

EPCLUSA (sofosbuvir/velpatasvir): antiviral; Rx: hepatitis C

Ephedrine: bronchodilator; Rx: asthma, COPD

EPIPEN (epinephrine): bronchodilator/vasoconstrictor; Rx: allergic reaction

EPIVIR, EPIVIR HBV (lamivudine): antiretroviral; Rx: HIV, hepatitis B

Epoetin alfa (EPOGEN): increases RBC production; Rx: anemia

EPOGEN (epoetin alfa): increases RBC production; Rx: anemia

Eptinezumab-jjmr (VYEPTI): antimigraine; Rx: migraine prevention

EPZICOM (abacavir/lamivudine): antiretroviral; Rx: HIV

EQUETRO (carbamazepine): anticonvulsant; Rx: bipolar disorder

Erenumab-aooe (AIMOVIG): antimigraine; Rx: migraine prevention

Ergocalciferol (CALCIFEROL): vitamin D; Rx: hypocalcemia, hypoparathyroidism, rickets, osteodystrophy

Ertugliflozin (STEGLATRO): antidiabetic; Rx: Type 2 diabetes

ERYPED (erythromycin): macrolide antibiotic; Rx: bacterial infection

ERY-TAB (erythromycin): antibiotic; Rx: bacterial infection

Erythromycin (E.E.S.): antibiotic; Rx: bacterial infection

ESGIC (acetaminophen/caffeine/butalbital): analgesic/muscle relaxant/antianxiety compound; Rx: headache

Estazolam: benzodiazepine, sedative/hypnotic; Rx: insomnia

ESTRACE (estradiol): estrogen; Rx: symptoms of menopause

Estropipate: estrogens; Rx: symptoms of menopause

Ethacrynic acid (EDECRIN): diuretic; Rx: pulmonary edema, HF

Ethambutol (MYAMBUTOL): Rx: pulmonary tuberculosis

Ethosuximide (ZARONTIN): anticonvulsant; Rx: absence Sz

Etodolac (LODINE): NSAID analgesic; Rx: arthritis

EVENITY (romosozumab-aqqg): monoclonal antibody; Rx: osteoporosis

EVISTA (raloxifene): estrogen modulator; Rx: osteoporosis, breast cancer prevention

Evolocumab (REPATHA): monoclonal antibody; Rx: hypercholesterolemia

EXELON (rivastigmine): cholinesterase inhibitor; Rx: dementia in Alzheimer's and Parkinson's disease

F

Famciclovir: antiviral; Rx: herpes

Famotidine (PEPCID): H-2 blocker, inhibits gastric acid; Rx: ulcers

FANAPT (iloperidone): antipsychotic; Rx: schizophrenia

FELBATOL (felbamate): antiepileptic; Rx: Sz

FELDENE (piroxicam): NSAID analgesic; Rx: arthrritis

Felodipine: calcium channel blocker; Rx: HTN

FEMARA (letrozole): estrogen inhibitor; Rx: breast cancer

Fenofibrate (TRICOR): lipid regulator; Rx: hyperlipidemia

Fentanyl: opioid analgesic; Rx: moderate-to-severe pain

FERRLECIT (sodium ferric gluconate complex): hematinic; Rx: iron deficiency anemia in hemodialysis

Fexofenadine (ALLEGRA): antihistamine; Rx: allergies

Finasteride (PROSCAR, PROPECIA): antiandrogen; Rx: hair loss, BPH

FIORICET (butalbital/acetaminophen/caffeine): sedative, analgesic; Rx: tension H/A

FIORINAL (butalbital/ASA/caffeine): sedative analgesic; Rx: tension H/A

FLAGYL (metronidazole): antibiotic; Rx: bacterial infections

Flecainide: antiarrhythmic; Rx: PSVT, paroxysmal atrial fibrillation

FLOMAX (tamsulosin): α-1 blocker; Rx: BPH

FLONASE (fluticasone): nasal corticosteroid; Rx: allergic rhinitis

FLOVENT HFA (fluticasone): inhaled corticosteroid; Rx: asthma

Fluconazole (DIFLUCAN): antifungal; Rx: yeast infection

FLUMADINE (rimantadine): antiviral; Rx: influenza A virus

Flumazenil (ROMAZICON): antidote; Rx: benzodiazepine overdose

Flunisolide: inhaled corticosteroid; Rx: asthma

Flunisolide: nasal corticosteroid; Rx: allergic rhinitis

Fluocinolone (SYNALAR): topical corticosteroid; Rx: dermatoses

Fluocinonide: topical corticosteroid; Rx: dermatoses

Fluoxetine (PROZAC): antidepressant; Rx: depression, obsessive-compulsive disorder, bulimia

Fluphenazine: antipsychotic; Rx: schizophrenia

Flurazepam: benzodiazepine; Rx: insomnia

Flurbiprofen: NSAID analgesic; Rx: arthritis

Flutamide (EULEXIN): antiandrogenic; Rx: prostate cancer

Fluticasone (CUTIVATE, FLONASE): steroid anti-inflammatory; Rx: dermatoses, asthma

Fluvastatin (LESCOL): statin; Rx: hypercholesterolemia

Fluvoxamine: SSRI; Rx: obsessive-compulsive disorder, anxiety

FOCALIN (dexmethylphenidate): stimulant; Rx: ADHD, NDRIs

FORTAZ (ceftazidime): cephalosporin antibiotic; Rx: bacterial infections

FOSAMAX (alendronate): reduces bone loss; Rx: osteoporosis, Paget's disease

Fosinopril: ACE inhibitor; Rx: HTN, HF

Fosphenytoin (CEREBYX): anticonvulsant; Rx: Sz

FOSRENOL (lanthanum): phosphate binder; Rx: hyperphosphatemia in ESRD

FRAGMIN (daltaparin): LMWH; Rx: prophylaxis/tx DVT/PE, ACS

Fremanezumab-vfrm (AJOVY): antimigraine; Rx: migraine prevention

FROVA (frovatriptan): serotonin receptor agonist; Rx: migraine headaches

Furosemide (LASIX): loop diuretic; Rx: HF, hypertension

FUZEON (enfuvirtide): antiretroviral; Rx: HIV

G

Gabapentin (NEURONTIN): anticonvulsant; Rx: Sz, persistent pain

GABITRIL (tiagabine): anticonvulsant; Rx: partial Sz

Galantamine: cholinergic enhancer; Rx: Alzheimer's disease

Galcanezumab-gnlm (EMGALITY): antimigraine; Rx: migraine prevention

Ganciclovir (CYTOVENE): antiviral; Rx: CMV

Gemfibrozil (LOPID): antihyperlipidemic; Rx: hypertriglyceridemia

GEMTESA (vibegron): β-3 agonist; Rx: overactive bladder

GENGRAF (cyclosporine): immunosuppressive; Rx: rheumatoid arthritis, psoriasis, prevention of transplant rejection

Gentamicin (GARAMYCIN): aminoglycoside antibiotic; Rx: bacterial infections

GEODON (ziprasidone): antipsychotic; Rx: schizophrenia

GLEEVEC (imatinib): antineoplastic, kinase inhibitor; Rx: leukemia, gastrointestinal cancer

Glimepiride (AMARYL): oral hypoglycemic; Rx: diabetes

Glipizide (GLUCOTROL): oral hypoglycemic; Rx: diabetes

Glucagon: hormone, mobilizes glucose; Rx: hypoglycemia

GLUCOTROL (glipizide): oral hypoglycemic; Rx: diabetes

Glyburide (GLYNASE): oral hypoglycemic; Rx: diabetes

Glycopyrrolate (ROBINUL): anticholinergic; Rx: peptic ulcers

GLYNASE (glyburide): oral hypoglycemic; Rx: diabetes

GLYSET (miglitol): alpha-glucosidase inhibitor, oral hypoglycemic; Rx: diabetes

Granisetron: antiemetic; Rx: chemotherapy-induced N/V

Griseofulvin: antifungal; Rx: ringworm, onychomycosis

Guaifenesin (HUMIBID, MUCINEX): expectorant; Rx: loosen bronchial secretions

Guanfacine: α-2 agonist, antihypertensive; Rx: HTN

H

HALCION (triazolam): benzodiazepine hypnotic; Rx: insomnia

Halobetasol (ULTRAVATE): topical corticosteroid; Rx: dermatoses

Haloperidol: antipsychotic; Rx: schizophrenia, psychotic disorders

HCT, HCTZ (hydrochlorothiazide): diuretic; Rx: HTN, water retention

Histex (triprolidine): antihistamine/decongestant; Rx: allergies, hay fever, cold

HUMALOG (insulin lispro): hypoglycemic; Rx: diabetes

HUMIBID (guaifenesin): expectorant; Rx: loosen bronchial secretions

HUMIRA (adalimumab): immunomodulator; Rx: rheumatoid and psoriatic arthritis, ankylosing spondylitis, Crohn's disease, IBD, TNF inhibitors

HUMULIN R (regular insulin): hypoglycemic; Rx: diabetes

HYCODAN (hydrocodone/homatropine): narcotic antitussive, anticholinergic, opioid

Hydralazine: vasodilator; Rx: HTN, HF

Hydrochlorothiazide (HCTZ): thiazide diuretic; Rx: HTN, water retention

Hydrocodone/acetaminophen (LORTAB): narcotic analgesic compound; Rx: moderate-to-severe pain

Hydrocortisone (CORTEF): topical corticosteroid; Rx: dermatoses

Hydromorphone (DILAUDID): opioid analgesic; Rx: moderate-to-severe pain

Hydroxychloroquine (PLAQUENIL): antimalarial; Rx: malaria, lupus, rheumatoid arthritis

Hydroxyurea (DROXIA, HYDREA): antineoplastic, elastogenic; Rx: melanoma, leukemia, ovarian cancer, sickle cell anemia

Hydroxyzine (VISTARIL): antihistamine; Rx: allergies, anxiety, sedation

Hyoscyamine (LEVSIN): antispasmodic; Rx: lower urinary tract and GI tract spasm/secretions

HYZAAR (losartan/HCTZ): thiazide diuretic, angiotensin receptor blocker; Rx: HTN

I

Ibutilide (CORVERT): antiarrhythmic; Rx: AF, atrial flutter

Imipenem/cilastatin (PRIMAXIN): carbapenem antibiotic; Rx: bacterial infections

Imipramine (TOFRANIL): tricyclic antidepressant; Rx: depression, bed wetting

IMITREX (sumatriptan): selective serotonin receptor agonist; Rx: migraine H/A

IMODIUM (loperamide): slows peristalsis; Rx: diarrhea

IMURAN (azathioprine): immunosuppressant; Rx: organ transplants, lupus, rheumatoid arthritis

Indapamide: diuretic; Rx: HTN, edema in HF

INDERAL, INDERAL LA (propranolol): β blocker; Rx: HTN, angina, cardiac dysrhythmias, AMI, migraine H/A

INDOCIN, INDOCIN SR (indomethacin): NSAID analgesic; Rx: arthritis

Indomethacin (INDOCIN): NSAID analgesic; Rx: arthritis

INFERGEN (interferon alfacon-1): antiviral; Rx: hepatitis C

Infliximab (REMICADE): neutralizes tumor necrosis factor; Rx: Crohn's disease

INH (isoniazid): antibiotic; Rx: tuberculosis

INSPRA (eplerenone): aldosterone blocker; Rx: HTN, HF

Insulin degludec (TRESIBA): long-acting insulin; Rx: diabetes

INTELENCE (etravirine): antiretroviral; Rx: HIV

INVEGA (paliperidone): antipsychotic; Rx: schizophrenia

Ipecac: detoxification agent; Rx: overdose/poisoning

Ipratropium (ATROVENT): bronchodilator; Rx: COPD

Irinotecan (CAMPTOSAR): antineoplastic; Rx: colon and rectal cancer

ISENTRESS (raltegravir): antiretroviral; Rx: HIV

Isoniazid: antibiotic; Rx: tuberculosis

Isoproterenol: β-bronchodilator; Rx: asthma, COPD

Isradipine: calcium channel blocker; Rx: HTN

Itraconazole (SPORANOX): antifungal; Rx: fungal infections

J

JANUMET (sitagliptin/metformin): oral hypoglycemics; Rx: diabetes

JANUVIA (sitagliptin): oral hypoglycemic; Rx: diabetes

K

KALETRA (lopinavir/ritonavir): antiretrovirals; Rx: HIV

KAOPECTATE (bismuth): gastrointestinal; Rx: indigestion, diarrhea

KAYEXALATE (sodium polysterene sulfonate): Na/K exchange resin; Rx: hyperkalemia

K-DUR (potassium): electrolyte; Rx: hypokalemia

KEPPRA (levatiracetam): anticonvulsant; Rx: Sz

Ketoconazole: antifungal agent; Rx: fungal infections

Ketoprofen: NSAID analgesic; Rx: arthritis

Ketorolac: NSAID analgesic; Rx: acute pain

KEVZARA (sarilumab): antirheumatic; Rx: rheumatoid arthritis

KLONOPIN (clonazepam): benzodiazepine hypnotic; Rx: seizures, panic disorder

KLOR-CON (potassium): electrolyte; Rx: hypokalemia

L

Labetalol: β-blocker; Rx: HTN

LACRI-LUBE OPTH (white petrolatum/mineral oil): Rx: ophthalmic lubrication

Lactulose: hyperosmotic laxative; Rx: constipation, encephalopathy

LAMICTAL (lamotrigine): anticonvulsant; Rx: Sz, bipolar disorder

Lamivudine (EPIVIR): antiviral; Rx: HIV

Lamotrigine (LAMICTAL): anticonvulsant; Rx: Sz, bipolar disorder

LANOXIN (digoxin): cardiac glycoside; Rx: HF, atrial fibrillation

Lansoprazole (PREVACID): gastric acid pump inhibitor; Rx: ulcers, GERD

LANTUS (insulin glargine): hypoglycemic; Rx: diabetes

LASIX (furosemide): loop diuretic; Rx: HTN, HF

Lasmiditan (REYVOW): antimigraine; Rx: migraine treatment

Latanoprost OPTH (XALATAN): F2α blocker; Rx: glaucoma

Leflunomide (ARAVA): immunomodulator, anti-inflammatory; Rx: rheumatoid arthritis

Lemborexant (DAYVIGO): hypnotic; Rx: insomnia

LESCOL (fluvastatin): statin; Rx: hypercholesterolemia

Leucovorin: vitamin; Rx: methotrexate toxicity, megaloblastic anemia

Leuprolide (LUPRON): hormone; Rx: endometriosis, advanced prostate cancer

Levalbuterol (XOPENEX): inhaled β-2 bronchodilator; Rx: COPD, asthma

Levatiracetam (KEPPRA): anticonvulsant; Rx: Sz

LEVEMIR (insulin detemir): hypoglycemic; Rx: diabetes

Levobunolol OPTH: β-blocker; Rx: glaucoma

Levodopa/carbidopa (SINEMET): dopamine precursor; Rx: Parkinson's disease

Levofloxacin: fluoroquinolone antibiotic; Rx: bacterial infections

LEVORA (levonorgestrel/estradiol): oral contraceptive

Levothyroxine (LEVOXYL, SYNTHROID): thyroid hormone; Rx: hypothyroidism

LEVOXYL (levothyroxine): thyroid hormone; Rx: hypothyroidism

LEXAPRO (escitalopram): SSRI antidepressant; Rx: depression, anxiety disorder

LEXIVA (fosamprenavir): antiretroviral; Rx: HIV

LIDODERM (lidocaine) topical local anesthetic; Rx: postherpetic neuralgia

Lindane: parasiticide; Rx: scabies, lice

Liothyronine (CYTOMEL): thyroid hormone; Rx: hypothyroidism

Liotrix (THYROLAR): thyroid hormone; Rx: hypothyroidism

LIPITOR (atorvastatin): statin; Rx: hypercholesterolemia, HF

Lisinopril (ZESTRIL): ACE inhibitor; Rx: HTN, HF, AMI

Lisinopril/HCTZ (ZESTORETIC): ACE inhibitor; Rx: HTN, HF, AMI

Lithium (LITHOBID): antipsychotic; Rx: bipolar disorder

LITHOBID (lithium): antipsychotic; Rx: bipolar disorder

Lixisenatide (ADLYXIN): antidiabetic; Rx: diabetes

LOCOID (hydrocortisone): topical corticosteroid; Rx: dermatoses, seborrheic dermatitis

LOESTRIN (ethinyl estradiol/norethindrone): oral contraceptive

Lofexidine (LUCEMYRA): α-2 agonist; Rx: opioid withdrawal

LOMOTIL (diphenoxylate/atropine): opioid congener; Rx: diarrhea

LO/OVRAL (ethinyl estradiol/norgestrel): oral contraceptive

Loperamide (IMODIUM): slows peristalsis; Rx: diarrhea

LOPID (gemfibrozil): antihyperlipidemic; Rx: hypertriglyceridemia

Lopinavir/ritonavir (KALETRA): antiviral; Rx: HIV, AIDS

LOPRESSOR (metoprolol): β-1 blocker; Rx: hypertension

LOPROX (ciclopirox): antifungal; Rx: ringworm, candida

Loratadine (CLARITIN): antihistamine; Rx: allergies

Lorazepam (ATIVAN): benzodiazepine hypnotic; Rx: anxiety, status epilepticus

LORTAB (hydrocodone/acetaminophen): narcotic analgesic

Losartan (COZAAR): angiotensin receptor blocker; Rx: HTN, diabetic nephropathy

LOTENSIN (benazepril): ACE inhibitor; Rx: HTN, HF

LOTENSIN HCT (benazepril/HCTZ): ACE inhibitor/diuretic; Rx: HTN

LOTREL (amlodipine/benazepril): calcium channel blocker/ACE inhibitor; Rx: HTN

LOTRIMIN (clotrimazole): topical antifungal agent; Rx: fungal infections

LOTRONEX (alosetron): antidiarrheal; Rx: irritable bowel syndrome

Lovastatin (ALTOPREV): statin; Rx: hypercholesterolemia, HF

LOVENOX (enoxaparin): antigoagulant; Rx: prophylaxis/tx DVT/PE, ACS

Loxapine: antipsychotic; Rx: schizophrenia

LUCEMYRA (lofexidine): α-2 agonist; Rx: opioid withdrawal

LUCENTIS (ranibizumab): blood vessel growth inhibitor; Rx: macular degeneration

Lumateperone tosylate (CAPLYTA): antipsychotic; Rx: schizophremia

LUNESTA (eszopiclone): sedative; Rx: insomnia

LUPRON DEPOT (leuprolide): hormone; Rx: endometriosis, prostate cancer

LUPKYNIS (voclosporin): immunosuppressant; Rx: lupus nephritis

LYRICA (pregabalin): anticonvulsant; Rx: partial seizures, neuropathic pain

M

MACROBID (nitrofurantoin): nitrofuran antibiotic; Rx: UTI

MACRODANTIN (nitrofurantoin): nitrofuran antibiotic; Rx: UTI

Mafenide (SULFAMYLON): topical antimicrobial; Rx: burn wounds

MALARONE (atovaquone/proquanil): antimalarial agents; Rx: malaria prevention/tx

Malathion (OVIDE): organophosphate insecticide; Rx: head lice

Mannitol (OSMITROL): osmotic diuretic; Rx: cerebral edema, ICP

Maprotiline: tetracyclic antidepressant; Rx: depression, bipolar disorder, anxiety

MARINOL (dronabinol): appetite stimulant; Rx: weight loss in cancer, AIDS

MAVIK (trandolapril): ACE inhibitor; Rx: HTN, HF post MI

MAXALT (rizatriptan): selective serotonin receptor agonist; Rx: migraine headaches

MAXZIDE (triamterene/HCTZ): diuretics; Rx: HTN, water retention

Mebendazole (EMVERM): anthelmintic; Rx: intestinal worms

Meclizine (ANTIVERT): antinauseant; Rx: motion sickness

Meclofenamate: NSAID analgesic; Rx: arthritis, acute pain

MEDROL (methylprednisolone): glucocorticoid; Rx: adrenal insufficiency, allergies, rheumatoid arthritis

Medroxyprogesterone (PROVERA): progestin hormone; Rx: endometriosis, amenorrhea, uterine bleeding

Mefloquine: antimalarial; Rx: prevention and Tx of malaria

Megestrol: progestin, appetite stimulant; Rx: anorexia with AIDS; antineoplastic; cancer

Meloxicam: NSAID analgesic; Rx: arthritis

Meperidine (DEMEROL): opioid analgesic; Rx: moderate-to-severe pain

MEPHYTON (vitamin K1): Rx: coagulation disorders

MEPRON (atovaquone): antiprotozoal; Rx: prophylaxis and treatment for PCP in AIDS

Meropenem: carbapenem antibiotic; Rx: bacterial infections

Mesalamine (ASACOL, PENTASA): anti-inflammatory agent; Rx: ulcerative colitis

Metaproterenol: β-2 agonist bronchodilator; Rx: COPD, asthma

Metformin: oral hypoglycemic; Rx: diabetes

Methadone: opioid analgesic; Rx: moderate-to-severe pain, opiate withdrawal

METHADOSE (methadone): opioid analgesic; Rx: detoxification of opioid addiction

Methenamine: antibiotic; Rx: UTI prophylaxis

METHERGINE (methylergonovine): increases uterine contractions; Rx: uterine contraction/bleeding

Methimazole: antithyroid; Rx: hyperthyroidism

Methocarbamol (ROBAXIN): skeletal muscle relaxant

Methotrexate: antineoplastic; Rx: psoriasis, cancer, rheumatoid arthritis

Methsuximide: anticonvulsant; Rx: absence Sz

Methyldopa: centrally acting antihypertensive; Rx: HTN

Methylphenidate (RITALIN): stimulant; Rx: ADHD, narcolepsy

Methylprednisolone (MEDROL): glucocorticoid; Rx: adrenal insufficiency, allergies, RA

Metoclopramide (REGLAN): improves gastric emptying; Rx: heartburn, diabetic gastroparesis

Metolazone: thiazide diuretic; Rx: HTN, fluid retention

Metoprolol (LOPRESSOR, TOPROL-XL): β-1 blocker; Rx: HTN, angina, dysrhythmias

Metronidazole (FLAGYL): antibiotic; Rx: bacterial infections

Mexiletine: antiarrhythmic; Rx: ventricular dysrhythmias

MIACALCIN (calcitonin-salmon): bone resorption inhibitor hormone; Rx: hypercalcemia, Paget's disease, osteoporosis

MICARDIS (telmisartan): angiotensin II receptor antagonist; Rx: HTN

Miconazole (MONISTAT): antifungal; Rx: candidiasis

Midazolam: benzodiazepine hypnotic; Rx: anxiety before surgery

Midodrine: vasopressor; Rx: orthostatic hypotension

MINIPRESS (prazosin): α-1 blocker; Rx: hypertension

MINOCIN (minocycline): tetracycline antibiotic; Rx: bacterial infections, acne

Minocycline (MINOCIN): tetracycline antibiotic; Rx: bacterial infections, acne

Minoxidil: vasodilator; Rx: severe HTN

MIRALAX (polyethylene glycol): osmotic laxative; Rx: constipation

Mirtazapine (REMERON): antidepressant; Rx: depression

Misoprostol (CYTOTEC): antiulcer; Rx: NSAID-induced gastric ulcers

Modafinil (PROVIGIL): wakefulness-promoting agent; Rx: narcolepsy, daytime sleepiness

Moexipril: ACE inhibitor; Rx: HTN

Mometasone: nasal corticosteroid; Rx: allergic rhinitis

MOTEGRITY (prucalopride): GI agent (prokinetic); Rx: chronic constipation

MONUROL (fosfomycin): antibiotic; Rx: UTI

Morphine sulfate (MS CONTIN): opioid analgesic; Rx: moderate-to-severe pain

MOTOFEN (difenoxin/atropine): decreases intestinal motility; Rx: diarrhea

Moxifloxacin: fluoroquinolone antibiotic; Rx: bacterial infections

MS CONTIN (morphine ER): narcotic analgesic; Rx: moderate-to-severe pain

MUCINEX (guaifenesin): expectorant; Rx: loosen bronchial secretions

Mupirocin: topical antibiotic; Rx: skin infections

MYCOBUTIN (rifabutin): antibiotic; Rx: TB, *Mycobacterium avium* complex (MAC) in HIV

MYLERAN (busulfan): alkylating agent; Rx: leukemia

MYSOLINE (primidone): anticonvulsant; Rx: Sz

N

Nabumetone: NSAID analgesic; Rx: arthritis

Nadolol (CORGARD): β-blocker; Rx: HTN, angina

Nafcillin: penicillin antibiotic; Rx: bacterial infection

Nalbuphine: opioid agonist-antagonist analgesic; Rx: pain relief, pruritus

Naltrexone/bupropion (CONTRAVE): antidepressant; Rx: weight management

NAMENDA (memantine): NMDA antagonist; Rx: Alzheimer's disease

NAPROSYN (naproxen): NSAID analgesic; Rx: arthritis, pain, inflammation, H/A

NARDIL (phenelzine): MAO inhibitor; Rx: depression, bulimia

NASALCROM (cromolyn): nasal anti-inflammatory agent; Rx: allergic rhinitis

Nefazodone: antidepressant; Rx: depression

Nelfinavir (VIRACEPT): protease inhibitor antiretroviral; Rx: HIV

NEMBUTAL (pentobarbital): barbiturate; Rx: insomnia, sleep induction, status epilepticus

NEOSPORIN (neomycin/polymyxin/bacitracin): topical antibiotic compound; Rx: topical infections

NEUPOGEN (filgrastim): white blood cell stimulator; Rx: chemotherapy, bone marrow transplant

NEURONTIN (gabapentin): anticonvulsant; Rx: Sz, persistent pain

Nevirapine: antiretroviral; Rx: HIV

NEXIUM (esomeprazole): protein pump inhibitor; Rx: esophagitis, GERD, ulcers

Niacin (vitamin B3): nicotinic acid; Rx: hypercholesterolemia, hypertriglyceridemia

NIACOR (niacin): vitamin B3; Rx: hypercholesterolemia, hypertriglyceridemia

Nicardipine (CARDENE): calcium channel blocker; Rx: angina, HTN

NICODERM (transdermal nicotine): Rx: smoking cessation

Nicotinic acid (niacin): vitamin B3; Rx: hypercholesterolemia, hypertriglyceridemia

NICOTROL inhaler (nicotine): Rx: smoking cessation

NICOTROL NS (nicotine): Rx: smoking cessation

Nifedipine: calcium channel blocker; Rx: angina, HTN

NILANDRON (nilutamide): antiandrogen; Rx: prostate cancer

Nimodipine: calcium channel blocker; Rx: improves neurologic deficits after subarachnoid hemorrhage

Nisoldipine (SULAR): calcium channel blocker; Rx: HTN

NITRO-DUR (nitroglycerin): transdermal nitrate; Rx: angina

Nitrofurantoin (macrodantin): antibacterial agent; Rx: UTI

Nitroglycerin (NITROSTAT): vasodilator; Rx: angina

NITROLINGUAL SPRAY (nitroglycerin): nitrate; Rx: angina

NITROMIST (nitroglycerin): vasodilator lingual spray; Rx: angina

NITROSTAT (nitroglycerin): vasodilator; Rx: angina

Nizatidine: histamine-2 antagonist; Rx: ulcers, GERD

Norfloxacin: fluoroquinolone antibiotic; Rx: bacterial infections

NORGESIC (orphenadrine): skeletal muscle relaxant

NORPACE, NORPACE CR (disopyramide): antiarrhythmic; Rx: ventricular dysrhythmias

NORPRAMIN (desipramine): tricyclic antidepressant; Rx: depression

Nortriptyline (PAMELOR): tricyclic antidepressant; Rx: depression

NORVASC (amlodipine): calcium blocker; Rx: HTN, angina

NORVIR (ritonavir): protease inhibitor antiretroviral; Rx: HIV

NOVOLIN R (regular insulin): hypoglycemic; Rx: diabetes

NOVOLOG (insulin aspart): hypoglycemic; Rx: diabetes

NOVOLOG MIX 70/30 (insulin mixture): hypoglycemic; Rx: diabetes

NURTEC ODT (rimegepant): antimigraine agent; Rx: migraine treatment

NUVIGIL (armodafinil): CNS stimulant; Rx: narcolepsy, shift-work sleep disorder

Nystatin: antifungal; Rx: candidiasis

NYSTOP (nystatin): antifungal; Rx: candidiasis

O

Olanzapine (ZYPREXA): antipsychotic; Rx: schizophrenia, bipolar disorder

Olopatadine: antihistamine; Rx: allergic conjunctivitis

OLUMIANT (baricitinib): antirheumatic; Rx: rheumatoid arthritis

Olsalazine (DIPENTUM): salicylate; Rx: ulcerative colitis

Omeprazole (PRILOSEC): suppresses gastric acid secretion; Rx: ulcers, esophagitis, GERD

OMNARIS (ciclesonide): intranasal steroid; Rx: allergic rhinitis

Ondansetron (ZOFRAN): antinauseant; Rx: N/V secondary to chemotherapy, radiation, and surgery

ONGENTYS (opicapone): antiparkinson agent; Rx: Parkinson's

Opicapone (ONGENTYS): antiparkinson agent; Rx: Parkinson's

Opium tincture (morphine): opioid analgesic; Rx: diarrhea

ORAMORPH SR (morphine sulfate SR): opioid analgesic; Rx: moderate-to-severe pain

ORENCIA (abatacept): immunomodulator; Rx: rheumatoid arthritis

ORGOVYX (relugolix): chemotherapeutic; Rx: prostate cancer

Orphenadrine: skeletal muscle relaxant

Oxacillin: penicillin class antibiotic; Rx: bacterial infections

Oxandrolone: anabolic steroid; Rx: osteoporosis, promotes weight gain

Oxaprozin (DAYPRO): NSAID analgesic; Rx: arthritis

Oxazepam: benzodiazepine hypnotic; Rx: anxiety, alcohol withdrawal

Oxcarbazepine (TRILEPTAL): anticonvulsant; Rx: partial Sz

Oxybutynin (DITROPAN): anticholinergic, antispasmodic; Rx: overactive bladder

Oxycodone (ROXICODONE, OXYCONTIN): opioid analgesic; Rx: moderate-to-severe pain

Oxycodone/ASA: opioid analgesic/aspirin; Rx: moderate-to-severe pain

Oxycodone with acetaminophen (ENDOCET, PERCOCET): opioid analgesic/acetaminophen; Rx: moderate-to-severe pain

OXYCONTIN (oxycodone SR): opioid analgesic; Rx: moderate-to-severe pain

Oxymetazoline (AFRIN): nasal decongestant; Rx: sinusitis, cold

Oxymetholone: anabolic steroid/androgen; Rx: anemia

Oxymorphone: opioid analgesic; Rx: moderate-to-severe pain

Oxytocin (PITOCIN): stimulates uterine contractions; Rx: induction of labor

OXYTROL (oxybutynin): transdermal anticholinergic, antispasmodic; Rx: overactive bladder

OZEMPIC (semaglutide): antidiabetic; Rx: type 2 diabetes

P

PACERONE (amiodarone): antiarrhythmic; Rx: dysrhythmias

PAMELOR (nortriptyline): tricyclic antidepressant; Rx: depression

Pantoprazole (PROTONIX): suppresses gastic acid; Rx: ulcers, GERD

PARCOPA (carbidopa/levodopa): dopamine precursors; Rx: Parkinson's disease

PAREGORIC (morphine): opioid analgesic; Rx: diarrhea

Paricalcitol (ZEMPLAR): vitamin D; Rx: hyperparathyroidism in chronic kidney disease

PARNATE (tranylcypromine): MAO inhibitor; Rx: depression

Paroxetine (PAXIL): SSRI antidepressant; Rx: depression, OCD, anxiety, PTSD

PATANASE (olopatadine): nasal antihistamine; Rx: allergic rhinitis

PAXIL (paroxetine): SSRI antidepressant; Rx: depression, OCD, anxiety, PTSD

PEDIAPRED (prednisolone): glucocorticoid; Rx: allergies, arthritis, MS

Penciclovir (DENAVIR): topical antiviral; Rx: herpes, cold sores

Penicillin: antibiotic; Rx: bacterial infection

Pentamidine (PENTAM): antiprotozoal; Rx: PCP

PENTASA (mesalamine): anti-inflammatory; Rx: ulcerative colitis

Pentazocine: opioid agonist-antagonist analgesic; Rx: moderate-to-severe pain

Pentobarbital (NEMBUTAL): barbiturate hypnotic; Rx: insomnia, status epilepticus

Pentoxifylline: reduces blood viscosity; Rx: intermittent claudication

PEPCID, PEPCID AC (famotidine): H2 blocker reduces gastric acid; Rx: ulcers, GERD

PERCOCET (oxycodone/acetaminophen): opioid analgesic; Rx: moderate-to-severe pain

PERI-COLACE (docusate/senna): stool softener/laxative; Rx: constipation

Perindopril: ACE inhibitor; Rx: HTN, CAD

Permethrin: parasiticide; Rx: head lice, scabies

Perphenazine: antipsychotic; Rx: schizophrenia, hiccups

Phenazopyridine (PYRIDIUM): urinary tract analgesic; Rx: relief of pain on urination

Phenelzine (NARDIL): MAO inhibitor; Rx: depression

PHENERGAN (promethazine): sedative/antiemetic; Rx: rhinitis, urticaria, N&V

Phenobarbital: barbiturate sedative; Rx: sedative, anticonvulsant

Phenylephrine (SUDAFED PE): decongestant; Rx: colds, allergies

Phenytoin (DILANTIN): anticonvulsant; Rx: epilepsy

PHISOHEX (hexachlorophene): bacteriostatic skin cleanser

PhosLo (calcium): phosphate binder; Rx: hyperphosphatemia in ESRD

Phytonadione: vitamin K1; Rx: coagulation disorders

PIFELTRO (doravirine): antiretroviral; Rx: HIV infection

Pilocarpine (SALAGEN): cholinergic; Rx: dry mouth, Sjogren's syndrome

Pilocarpine OPTH: cholinergic miotic; Rx: glaucoma

Pindolol: β-blocker; Rx: HTN

Pioglitazone (ACTOS): oral hypoglycemic; Rx: diabetes

Piperacillin: penicillin antibiotic; Rx: bacterial infections

Piroxicam (FELDENE): NSAID analgesic; Rx: arthritis

Pitolisant (WAKIX): CNS stimulant; Rx: narcolepsy

PLAQUENIL (hydroxychloroquine): antimalarial agent; Rx: malaria, rheumatoid arthritis, lupus

PLAVIX (clopidogrel): platelet inhibitor; Rx: MI, stroke, atherosclerosis

Plazomicin (ZEMDRI): antibiotic; Rx: complicated UTIs

Polyethylene glycol (MIRALAX): osmotic laxative; Rx: constipation

Posaconazole (NOXAFIL): antifungal; Rx: fungal infections

Potassium citrate (UROCIT-K): urinary alkalinizer; Rx: kidney stones

PRALUENT (alirocumab): monoclonal antibody; Rx: hypercholesterolemia

Pramipexole: dopamine agonist; Rx: Parkinson's disease, restless legs syndrome

Pravastatin: statin; Rx: hypercholesterolemia, CAD

Prazosin (MINIPRESS): α-1 blocker, vasodilator; Rx: HTN

Prednisolone: glucocorticoid; Rx: adrenal insufficiency, allergies, rheumatoid arthritis, lupus, COPD

Prednisone: glucocorticoid; Rx: adrenal insufficiency, allergies, RA, lupus, COPD

PREMARIN (conjugated estrogens): hormone; Rx: menopause

PREMPRO (estrogens/progesterone): hormone; Rx: menopause

Drugs

PREVACID (lansoprazole): gastric acid pump inhibitor; Rx: ulcers, esophagitis, GERD

PREVPAC (lansoprazole/amoxicillin/clarithromycin): *H. pylori* treatment; Rx: duodenal ulcers

PRIFTIN (rifapentine): antibiotic; Rx: tuberculosis

PRILOSEC (omeprazole): gastric acid pump inhibitor; Rx: ulcers, esophagitis, GERD

Primaquine: antimalarial agent; Rx: malaria

Primidone (MYSOLINE): anticonvulsant; Rx: Sz

PRISTIQ (desvenlafaxine): antidepressant; Rx: depression

Probenecid: increases uric acid secretion; Rx: gout

Procainamide: antiarrhythmic; Rx: dysrhythmias

Prochlorperazine: phenothiazine antiemetic; Rx: N/V, anxiety

PROCRIT (epoetin alfa): stimulates red blood cell production; Rx: anemia, renal failure, HIV, chemotherapy

Progesterone (PROMETRIUM): progestin; Rx: endometrial hyperplasia, secondary amenorrhea

PROGRAF (tacrolimus): immunosuppressant; Rx: transplant

PROLASTIN (α-1 proteinase inhibitor): Rx: α-PI antitrypsin deficiency, emphysema

Promethazine (PHENERGAN): phenothiazine; Rx: rhinitis, allergic conjunctivitis, sedation, N/V

PROMETRIUM (progesterone): progestin; Rx: endometrial hyperplasia, secondary amenorrhea

Propafenone (RYTHMOL): β-blocker, antiarrhythmic; Rx: PSVT, paroxysmal atrial fibrillation

Propantheline: anticholinergic, inhibits gastric acid secretion; Rx: peptic ulcers

Proparacaine OPTH (ALCAINE): anesthetic; Rx: corneal anesthesia

Propranolol (INDERAL): β-blocker; Rx: HTN; prophylaxis of angina, cardiac dysrhythmias, AMI, migraine H/A

Propylthiouracil: antithyroid; Rx: hyperthyroidism

PROSCAR (finasteride): antiandrogen; Rx: benign prostatic hypertrophy

PROTONIX (pantoprazole): proton pump inhibitor; Rx: ulcers, GERD

PROVENTIL, PROVENTIL HFA (albuterol): β-2 agonist bronchodilator; Rx: COPD, asthma

PROVERA (medroxyprogesterone): hormone, progesterone; Rx: amenorrhea, irregular vaginal bleeding, endometrial or renal cancer

PROVIGIL (modafinil): stimulant; Rx: narcolepsy, daytime sleepiness

PROZAC (fluoxetine): SSRI antidepressant

Prucalopride (MOTEGRITY): GI agent (prokinetic); Rx: chronic constipation

Pseudoephedrine (SUDAFED): decongestant; Rx: colds, allergies

Psyllium (METAMUCIL): fiber laxative; Rx: constipation

PULMOZYME (dornase alfa): lytic enzyme, dissolves lung secretions; Rx: cystic fibrosis

Pyrazinamide: antibacterial; Rx: tuberculosis

PYRIDIUM (phenazopyridine): urinary tract analgesic; Rx: relief of pain on urination

Pyridostigmine (MESTINON): anticholinesterase; Rx: myasthenia gravis

Pyridoxine: vitamin B6

Pyrimethamine (DARAPRIM): antiparasitic; Rx: toxoplasmosis, malaria

Q

QUALAQUIN (quinine): antimalarial; Rx: malaria

QUESTRAN (cholestyramine): bile acid sequestrant; Rx: antihyperlipidemic

Quetiapine (SEROQUEL): antipsychotic; Rx: schizophrenia, bipolar disorder

Quinapril (ACCUPRIL): ACE inhibitor; Rx: HTN, HF

Quinapril/HCTZ (ACCURETIC): ACE inhibitor/diuretic; Rx: HTN

Quinine: antimalarial; Rx: malaria

R

Raloxifene (EVISTA): estrogen modulator; Rx: osteoporosis, breast cancer prevention

Ramipril (ALTACE): ACE inhibitor; Rx: HTN, HF post MI

Ranolazine: anti-ischemic; Rx: chronic angina

RAPAFLO (silodosin): α receptor agonist, Rx; BPH

RAPAMUNE (sirolimus): immunosuppressive; Rx: renal transplant

Rebif (interferon-β-1a): immunomodulator; Rx: multiple sclerosis

RECOMBINATE (Factor VIII): antihemophilic factor; Rx: hemophilia

REGLAN (metoclopramide): improves gastric emptying; Rx: heartburn, diabetic gastroparesis

RELENZA (zanamivir): antiviral; Rx: influenza

RELISTOR (methylnaltrexone): GI tract opioid antagonist; Rx: opioid-induced constipation

RELPAX (eletriptan): serotonin receptor agonist; Rx: migraine headaches

Relugolix (ORGOVYX): chemotherapeutic; Rx: prostate cancer

Remdesivir (VEKLURY): antiviral; Rx: COVID-19

REMERON (mirtazapine): antidepressant; Rx: depression

REMICADE (infliximab): neutralizes tumor necrosis factor; Rx: Crohn's disease, arthritis, ulcerative colitis, psoriasis

RENAGEL (sevelamer): phosphate binder; Rx: hyperphosphatemia in renal disease

REPATHA (evolocumab): monoclonal antibody; Rx: hypercholesterolemia

Reslizumab (CINQAIR): monoclonal antibody; Rx: severe asthma

RESTORIL (temazepam): benzodiazepine hypnotic; Rx: insomnia

RETIN A (tretinoin): retinoid; Rx: acne

RETROVIR (zidovudine): antiretroviral agent; Rx: HIV

REVATIO (sildenafil): vasodilator; Rx: pulmonary artery hypertension

Revefenacin (YUPELRI): long-acting bronchodilator; Rx: COPD

REXULTI (brexpiprazole): antipsychotic; Rx: schizophrenia

REYATAZ (atazanavir): antiretroviral; Rx: HIV

REYVOW (lasmiditan): antimigraine; Rx: migraine treatment

Ribavirin: antiviral; Rx: hepatitis C

RIFADIN (rifampin): antibiotic; Rx: tuberculosis, prophylaxis for *N. meningitidis*

Rifampin (RIFADIN): antibiotic; Rx: tuberculosis, prophylaxis for *N. meningitidis*

Rifamycin (AEMCOLO): antibiotic; Rx: travelers' diarrhea

Rifapentine (PRIFTIN): antibiotic; Rx: tuberculosis

Rifaximin (XIFAXAN): antibiotic; Rx: traveler's diarrhea, hepatic encephalopathy

Rimantadine (FLUMADINE): antiviral; Rx: influenza A virus

Rimegepant (NURTEC ODT): antimigraine agent; Rx: migraine treatment

RINVOQ (upadacitinib): antirheumatic; Rx: rheumatoid arthritis

RIOMET (metformin): oral hypoglycemic; Rx: diabetes

Risedronate (ACTONEL): bone stabilizer; Rx: Paget's disease, osteoporosis

RISPERDAL (risperidone): antipsychotic; Rx: schizophrenia, autism, bipolar disorder

Risperidone (RISPERDAL): antipsychotic; Rx: schizophrenia, autism, bipolar disorder

RITALIN (methylphenidate): stimulant; Rx: attention-deficit/hyperactivity disorder in children, narcolepsy

Ritonavir (NORVIR): antiretroviral; Rx: HIV

Rivastigmine (EXELON): cholinesterase inhibitor; Rx: dementia in Alzheimer's disease and Parkinson's disease

ROBAXIN (methocarbamol): skeletal muscle relaxant

ROBINUL FORTE (glycopyrrolate): anticholinergic; Rx: peptic ulcers

ROBITUSSIN (guaifenesin): expectorant

ROCALTROL (calcitrol): vitamin D analog; Rx: hypocalcemia in renal disease, hypoparathyroidism, bone disease

Romosozumab-aqqg (EVENITY): monoclonal antibody; Rx: osteoporosis

Ropinirole: dopaminergic; Rx: Parkinson's disease, restless leg syndrome

Rosiglitazone: oral hypoglycemic; Rx: diabetes

ROWASA (mesalamine): anti inflammatory; Rx: colitis, proctitis

ROXICODONE (oxycodone): opioid analgesic; Rx: moderate-to-severe pain

ROZEREM (ramelteon): melatonin agonist; Rx: insomnia
RYTHMOL, RYTHMOL SR (propafenone): antiarrhythmic; Rx: PSVT, paroxysmal atrial fibrillation

S

Sacubitril/valsartan (ENTRESTO): angiotensin II blocker; Rx: HF

Safinamide (XADAGO): antiparkinson agent; Rx: Parkinson's

SALAGEN (pilocarpine): cholinergic; Rx: dry mouth

Salmeterol (SEREVENT): inhaled β-2 agonist, bronchodilator; Rx: asthma, COPD

Salsalate: NSAID analgesic; Rx: arthritis

SANDIMMUNE (cyclosporine): immunosuppressant agent; Rx: organ transplants

SANDOSTATIN (octreotide): antidiarrheal, growth inhibitor; Rx: acromegaly, diarrhea associated with carcinoid and intestinal tumors

Sarilumab (KEVZARA): antirheumatic; Rx: rheumatoid arthritis

SAVAYSA (edoxaban): anticoagulant; Rx: AF

SAVELLA (milnacipran): selective serotonin/norepinephrine inhibitor; Rx: fibromyalgia

Scopolamine: anticholinergic; Rx: motion sickness, IBS, diverticulitis

Secobarbital: barbiturate hypnotic; Rx: insomnia

SECTRAL (acebutolol): β-blocker; Rx: HTN, angina, dysrhythmias

Selegiline: MAO inhibitor; Rx: Parkinson's disease

Semaglutide (OZEMPIC): antidiabetic; Rx: type 2 diabetes

SEMPREX-D (acrivastine/pseudoephedrine): antihistamine/decongestant; Rx: allergic rhinitis

Senna extract (SENOKOT): laxative; Rx: constipation

SENNA-S, SENOKOT-S (senna/docusate): laxative/stool softener; Rx: constipation

SENOKOT, SENOKOT XTRA (senna): laxative; Rx: constipation

SENSIPAR (cinacalcet): reduces PTH levels; Rx: hyperparathyroidism

SEREVENT (salmeterol): inhaled β-2 bronchodilator; Rx: asthma, COPD

SEROQUEL (quetiapine): antipsychotic; Rx: schizophrenia, bipolar disorder

SEROSTIM (somatropin): hormone; Rx: AIDS wasting

Sertraline (ZOLOFT): antidepressant; Rx: depression, panic disorder, obsessive-compulsive disorder, premenstrual dysphoric disorder

SILENOR (doxepin): TCA antidepressant; Rx: depression, insomnia

SILVADENE (silver sulfadiazine): topical antimicrobial agent; Rx: burn wounds

Simethicone (MYLICON): Rx: relief of excess gas in GI tract

Simvastatin (ZOCOR): statin; Rx: hypercholesterolemia, CAD

SINEMET CR (carbidopa/levodopa): dopamine precursors; Rx: Parkinson's disease

SINGULAIR (montelukast): leukotriene receptor antagonist; Rx: asthma, allergic rhinitis

Sirolimus (RAPAMUNE): immunosuppressive; Rx: renal transplant

SLO-NIACIN (niacin CR): vitamin B3; Rx: hypercholesterolemia, hypertriglyceridemia

Sodium polysterene sulfonate: Na/K exchange resin; Rx: hyperkalemia

Sofosbuvir/velpatasvir (EPCLUSA): antiviral; Rx: hepatitis C

Solriamfetol (SUNOSI): antiepileptic; Rx: narcolepsy

SOMA (carisoprodol): muscle relaxant; Rx: muscle spasm

Sotalol (BETAPACE): antiarrhythmic; Rx: dysrhythmias

SPECTRACEF (cefditoren): cephalosporin antibiotic; Rx: bacterial infections

SPIRIVA (tiotropium): inhaled anticholinergic bronchodilator; Rx: COPD

Spironolactone (ALDACTONE): potassium-sparing diuretic; Rx: hyperaldosteronism, HTN, HF

SPORANOX (itraconazole): antifungal; Rx: fungal infections

SSKI (potassium iodide): expectorant; Rx: asthma, bronchitis

STALEVO (levodopa/carbidopa/entacapone): dopamine precursors; Rx: Parkinson's disease

Stavudine d4T: antiretroviral; Rx: HIV

STEGLATRO (ertugliflozin): antidiabetic; Rx: type 2 diabetes

STRATTERA (atomoxetine): psychotherapeutic agent; Rx: ADHD

Streptomycin: aminoglycoside antibiotic; Rx: tuberculosis

STRIANT (testosterone): androgen; Rx: adult male hypogonadism

STROMECTOL (ivermectin): anti-parasite; Rx: parasites

SUBOXONE (buprenorphine/naloxone): opioid analgesic/antagonist; Rx: opiate addiction

Sucralfate (CARAFATE): antiulcer agent; Rx: duodenal ulcers

SULAR (nisoldipine): calcium channel blocker; Rx: HTN

Sulfamethoxazole: sulfa antibiotic; Rx: bacterial infections

Sulfasalazine (AZULFIDINE-EN-Tabs): anti-inflammatory; Rx: ulcerative colitis, rheumatoid arthritis

Sulfisoxazole: sulfonamide antibiotic; Rx: bacterial infections

Sulindac: NSAID analgesic; Rx: arthritis

Sumatriptan (IMITREX): selective serotonin receptor agonist; Rx: migraine H/A

SUNOSI (solriamfetol): antiepileptic; Rx: narcolepsy

SUPRAX (cefixime): cephalosporin antibiotic; Rx: bacterial infections

SURVANTA (beractant): lung surfactant in premature infants

SUSTIVA (efavirenz): antiretroviral; Rx: HIV

SYMBICORT (budesonide/formoterol): inhaled corticosteroid/β-2 agonist; Rx: asthma, COPD

SYMBYAX (olanzapine/fluoxetine) antipsychotic/SSRI; Rx: bipolar disorder, resistant depression

SYNAREL (naferelin): nasal gonadotropin-releasing hormone; Rx: endometriosis, precocious puberty

SYNTHROID (levothyroxine): thyroid hormone; Rx: hypothyroidism

T

TAGAMET HB (cimetidine): inhibits gastric acid secretion; Rx: ulcers

TAMIFLU (oseltamivir): antiviral; Rx: influenza

Tamoxifen: antiestrogen; Rx: breast cancer

TEGRETOL, TEGRETOL XR (carbamazepine): anticonvulsant; Rx: seizures, trigeminal neuralgia

TEKTURNA (Aliskeren): direct renin inhibitor; Rx: HTN

Telmisartan (MICARDIS): angiotensin II receptor agonist; Rx: HTN

Temazepam (RESTORIL): benzodiazepine hypnotic; Rx: insomnia

TENORMIN (atenolol): β blocker; Rx: HTN, angina, CAD

TENORETIC (atenolol/chlorthalidone): β-blocker/diuretic; Rx: HTN

Terazosin: α-1 blocker; Rx: HTN, benign prostatic hyperplasia

Terbinafine: antifungal; Rx: nail fungus, ringworm

Terbutaline: β-2 agonist bronchodilator; Rx: asthma, COPD

Terconazole (TERAZOL): antifungal; Rx: vaginal candidiasis

Testosterone (ANDRODERM, DEPO-TESTOSTERONE): androgen; Rx: hypogonadism

TESTRED (methyltestosterone): androgen; Rx: hypogonadism

Tetracycline: antibiotic; Rx: bacterial infections

TEVETEN (eprosartan): angiotensin II receptor inhibitor; Rx: HTN

Thalidomide (THALOMID): immunosuppressant; Rx: HIV, leprosy, multiple myeloma

THALOMID (thalidomide): immunosuppressant; Rx: HIV, leprosy, multiple myeloma

THEO-24 (theophylline): bronchodilator; Rx: asthma, COPD

Theophylline (THEO-24): bronchodilator; Rx: asthma, COPD

THERA-GESIC (salicylate): topical NSAID analgesic; Rx: arthritis

Thiamin: vitamin B1; Rx: thiamin deficiency

Thioridazine: antipsychotic; Rx: schizophrenia

Thiothixene: antipsychotic; Rx: schizophrenia

Thyroid (ARMOUR THYROID): thyroid hormone; Rx: hyporthyroidism

Tiagabine (GABITRIL): anticonvulsant; Rx: partial Sz

TIAZAC (diltiazem): calcium channel blocker; Rx: HTN, angina

Ticarcillin/clavulanate: penicillin antibiotic; Rx: bacterial infections

Ticlodipine: platelet inhibitor; Rx: stroke prophylaxis

TIGAN (trimethobenzamide): antiemetic; Rx: postoperative N/V

TIKOSYN (dofetilide): antiarrhythmic; Rx: AF

Timolol: β-blocker; Rx: HTN, MI, migraine

TIMOPTIC OPTH (timolol): β-blocker; Rx: glaucoma

TINACTIN (tolnaftate): topical antifungal; Rx: athlete's foot, jock itch

Tizanidine (ZANAFLEX): skeletal muscle relaxant

TOBI solution inhalation (tobramycin): aminoglycoside antibiotic; Rx: cystic fibrosis

Tobramycin (Tobrex OPTH): aminoglycoside antibiotic; Rx: bacterial infections

TOFRANIL, TOFRANIL PM (imipramine): tricyclic antidepressant; Rx: depression, anxiety

Tolazamide: oral hypoglycemic; Rx: diabetes

Tolbutamide: oral hypoglycemic; Rx: diabetes

Tolmetin: NSAID analgesic; Rx: arthritis

Tolnaftate (TINACTIN): topical antifungal; Rx: athlete's foot, jock itch

Tolterodine (DETROL): urinary bladder antispasmodic; Rx: overactive bladder

TOPAMAX (topiramate): anticonvulsant; Rx: seizures, migraine

TOPROL-XL (metoprolol): cardioselective β-blocker; Rx: HTN, angina, HF

Torsemide: loop diuretic; Rx: HTN, edema in HF, kidney disease, liver disease

TOVIAZ (fesoterodine): anticholinergic; Rx: overactive bladder

TRACLEER (bosentan): endothelin receptor antagonist; Rx: pulmonary hypertension

Tramadol: opioid analgesic; Rx: moderate-to-severe pain

Trandolapril (MAVIK): ACE inhibitor; Rx: HTN, HF post MI

TRANSDERM-SCOP (scopolamine): anticholinergic antiemetic; Rx: motion sickness prophylaxis

Trazodone: antidepressant; Rx: depression, insomnia

TRECATOR (ethionamide): antibiotic; Rx: tuberculosis

TRESIBA (insulin degludec): long-acting insulin; Rx: diabetes

Triamcinolone (KENALOG): steroid anti-inflammatory; Rx: dermatoses, asthma

Triamterenes/HCTZ (MAXZIDE): diuretics; Rx: HTN, water retention

Triazolam (HALCION): benzodiazepine hypnotic; Rx: insomnia

TRICOR (fenofibrate): lipid regulator; Rx: hyperlipidemia

Trifluoperazine: antipsychotic; Rx: schizophrenia

Trihexyphenidyl: anticholinergic; Rx: Parkinson's disease

TRILEPTAL (oxcarbazepine): anticonvulsant; Rx: partial Sz

Trimethoprim: antibiotic; Rx: UTI

Trimethoprim/sulfamethoxazole (BACTRIM): sulfa antibiotic compound; Rx: bacterial infections

TYKERB (lapatinib): antineoplastic; Rx: breast cancer

TRIZIVIR (abacavir/lamivudine/zidovudine): antiretrovirals; Rx: HIV infection, hepatitis B

TRUSOPT OPTH (dorzolamide): decreases intraocular pressure: Rx: glaucoma

TRUVADA (emtricitabine/tenofovir): antiretrovirals; Rx: HIV

TUSSIGON (hydrocodone/homatropine): narcotic antitussive, bronchodilator; Rx: cough

U

ULORIC (febuxostat): xanthine oxidase inhibitor; Rx: gout

UNISOM (doxylamine): antihistamine sedative; Rx: insomnia

Upadacitinib (RINVOQ): antirheumatic; Rx: rheumatoid arthritis

UROXATRAL (alfuzosin): smooth muscle relaxant; Rx: BPH

UROCIT-K (potassium citrate): urinary alkalinizer; Rx: kidney stones

Ursodiol: bile acid; Rx: gallstones

V

Valacyclovir (VALTREX): antiviral; Rx: herpes, shingles

VALCYTE (valganciclovir): antiviral; Rx: CMV

VALIUM (diazepam): benzodiazepine hypnotic; Rx: anxiety, muscle spasms, Sz, alcohol withdrawal

Valproic acid: anticonvulsant; Rx: Sz, migraines, mania

Valsartan (DIOVAN): angiotensin II receptor inhibitor; Rx: HTN, HF post-MI

VALTREX (valacyclovir): antiviral; Rx: herpes, shingles

VANCOCIN (vancomycin): antibiotic; Rx: bacterial infections

Vancomycin (VANCOCIN): antibiotic; Rx: bacterial infections

VASERETIC (enalapril/HCTZ): ACE inhibitor/diuretic; Rx: HTN

VASOTEC (enalapril): ACE inhibitor; Rx: HTN, HF

VEKLURY (remdesivir): antiviral; Rx: COVID-19

Venlafaxine (EFFEXOR): antidepressant; Rx: depression, anxiety, panic disorder

VENTOLIN HFA (albuterol): β-2 agonist bronchodilator; Rx: asthma, COPD

VERELAN, VERELAN PM (verapamil): calcium channel blocker; Rx: angina, hypertension, PSVT

VESICARE (solifenacin): anticholinergic; Rx: overactive bladder

VIAGRA (sildenafil): vasodilator; Rx: erectile dysfunction

Vibegron (GEMTESA): β-3 agonist; Rx: overactive bladder

VIBERZI (eluxadoline): GI agent; Rx: irritable bowel syndrome

VIBRAMYCIN (doxycycline): tetracycline antibiotic; Rx: bacterial infections

VIMPAT (lacosamide): anticonvulsant; Rx: partial onset Sz

VIRACEPT (nelfinavir): antiretroviral; Rx: HIV

VIREAD (tenofovir): antiretroviral; Rx: HIV, hepatitis B

VISTARIL (hydroxyzine): antihistamine; Rx: pruritus, sedation, anxiety

VIVELLE-DOT (estradiol): transdermal estrogen; Rx: symptoms of menopause

Voclosporin (LUPKYNIS): immunosuppressant; Rx: lupus nephritis

VRAYLAR (cariprazine): antipsychotic; Rx: schizophrenia and bipolar disorder

VYEPTI (eptinezumab-jjmr): antimigraine agent; Rx: migraine prevention

VYTORIN (ezetimibe/simvastatin): antihyperlipidemics; Rx: high cholesterol

W

WAKIX (pitolisant): CNS stimulant; Rx: narcolepsy
Warfarin: anticoagulant; Rx: AF, thrombosis
WELCHOL (colesevelam): bile acid sequestrant; Rx: hyperlipidemia
WELLBUTRIN SR (bupropion): antidepressant; Rx: depression

X

XADAGO (safinamide): antiparkinson agent; Rx: Parkinson's
XALATAN OPTH (latanoprost): reduces intraocular pressure; Rx: glaucoma
XANAX, XANAX XR (alprazolam): benzodiazepine; Rx: anxiety disorder, panic attacks
XELODA (capecitabine): antineoplastic; Rx: breast cancer, colorectal cancer
XENICAL (orlistat): lipase inhibitor; Rx: obesity
XIFAXAN (rifaximin): antibiotic; Rx: traveler's diarrhea, hepatic encephalopathy
XOFLUZA (baloxavir marboxil): antiviral; Rx: influenza
XOPENEX (levalbuterol): inhaled β-2 bronchodilator; Rx: asthma, COPD

Y

YASMIN 28 (drospirenone/estradiol): oral contraceptive
YAZ (drospirenone/estradiol): oral contraceptive
YUPELRI (revefenacin): long-acting bronchodilator; Rx: COPD

Z

Zaleplon: hypnotic; Rx: insomnia
ZANAFLEX (tizanidine): skeletal muscle relaxant
ZARONTIN (ethosuximide): anticonvulsant; Rx: absence Sz
ZEBETA (bisoprolol): β-blocker; Rx: HTN

ZEGERID (omeprazole/sodium bicarbonate): proton pump inhibitor compound; Rx: stress ulcer, ulcers, GERD

ZEMDRI (plazomicin): antibiotic; Rx: complicated UTIs

ZEMPLAR (paricalcitol): vitamin D analog; Rx: hyperparathyroidism in chronic kidney disease

ZESTORETIC (lisinopril/HCTZ): ACE inhibitor/diuretic; Rx: HTN

ZESTRIL (lisinopril): ACE inhibitor; Rx: HTN, HF

ZETIA (ezetimibe): antihyperlipidemic; Rx: hypercholesterolemia

ZIAGEN (abacavir): antiretroviral; Rx: HIV

Zidovudine (RETROVIR): antiretroviral; Rx: HIV

ZITHROMAX (azithromycin): macrolide antibiotic; Rx: bacterial infections

ZOCOR (simvastatin): statin; Rx: hypercholesterolemia, CAD

ZOFRAN (ondansetron): 5-HT3 receptor agonist; Rx: N/V due to chemotherapy, radiation, and surgery

ZOLADEX (goserelin): gonadotropin-releasing hormone agonist; Rx: endometriosis, prostate cancer, breast cancer

ZOLOFT (sertraline): antidepressant; Rx: depression, OCD, social anxiety disorder

Zolpidem (AMBIEN): hypnotic; Rx: insomnia

ZOMIG (zolmitriptan): serotonin receptor agonist; Rx: migraine H/A

ZONEGRAN (zonisamide): anticonvulsant; Rx: partial Sz

Zonisamide (ZONEGRAN): anticonvulsant; Rx: partial Sz

ZOVIRAX (acyclovir): antiviral; Rx: herpes, shingles, chickenpox

ZULRESSO (brexanolone): antidepressant; Rx: postpartum depression

ZYFLO (zileuton): bronchospasm inhibitor; Rx: asthma

ZYLOPRIM (allopurinol): xanthine oxidase inhibitor; Rx: gout

ZYPREXA, ZYPREXA ZYDIS (olanzapine): antipsychotic; Rx: schizophrenia, bipolar disorder

ZYRTEC (cetirizine): antihistamine; Rx: allergy, hives, asthma

ZYRTEC D (cetirizine/pseudoephedrine): antihistamine/decongestant; Rx: allergic rhinitis

ZYVOX (linezolid): oxazolidinone antibiotic; Rx: bacterial infections

Miscellaneous

1°	primary, first degree	ARC	AIDS-related complex
2°	secondary, second degree	asa	acetylsalicylic acid (aspirin)
3°	tertiary, third degree	ASAP	as soon as possible
α	alpha	ASHD	arteriosclerotic heart disease
@	at	ausc	auscultation
ā	before	AV	arteriovenous, atrioventricular
a.c., ac	before meals	ax	axillary
AAA	abdominal aortic aneurysm	β	beta
abd	abdomen	BBB	bundle branch block
ABG	arterial blood gas	b.i.d., bid	twice a day
abn	abnormal	bilat	bilateral
ADHD	attention deficit hyperactivity disorder	BM	bowel movement
adm.	administration	BP	blood pressure
AF	atrial fibrillation	BS	breath sounds
AIDS	acquired immune deficiency syndrome	BSA	body surface area
AKA	also known as	BSI	body substance isolation
AMA	against medical advice	BVM	bag-valve-mask
AMI	acute myocardial infarction	c̄	with
ANS	autonomic nervous system	C	centigrade
ant.	anterior	CABG	coronary artery bypass graft
A-P, AP	anterior-posterior	CAD	coronary artery disease
APAP	acetaminophen	CAO	conscious, alert, oriented
APE	acute pulmonary edema	CAT	computerized axial tomography

CBC	complete blood count	ECG	electrocardiogram
CC	chief complaint	EEG	electroencephalogram
CCU	coronary care unit	ED	emergency department
Cl	chloride	EENT	eyes, ears, nose, and throat
cm	centimeter	EMS	emergency medical services
CNS	central nervous system	ENT	ears, nose, and throat
c/o	complaining of	EPS	extrapyramidal symptoms (dystonias)
CO_2	carbon dioxide	ET	endotracheal
COHb	carboxyhemoglobin	$ETCO_2$	end-tidal carbon dioxide
COPD	chronic obstructive pulmonary disease	F	Fahrenheit
CPAP	continuous positive airway pressure	FH	family history
CSF	cerebrospinal fluid	FHR	fetal heart rate
CVA	cerebrovascular accident (stroke)	FUO	fever of undetermined origin
cx	chest	Fv	fever
D_5W	dextrose 5% in water	Fx	fracture
D/C	discontinue	g, gm	gram
DIC	disseminated intravascular coagulation	GCS	Glasgow coma scale
DKA	diabetic ketoacidosis	GI	gastrointestinal
dL	deciliter (100 mL)	gr	grain
DM	diabetes mellitus	GSW	gun shot wound
DMARD	disease-modifying antirheumatic drug	gtt	drops
DNR	do not resuscitate	GU	genitourinary
DOA	dead on arrival	GYN	gynecology
DOE	dyspnea on exertion	H/A	headache
DSD	dry sterile dressing	H&P	history and physical examination
DTR	deep tendon reflex	H+	hydrogen ion
DTs	delirium tremens	H_2O	water
Dx	diagnosis	Hb, Hgb	hemoglobin
EBL	estimated blood loss	HBP	high blood pressure

HCO₃⁻	bicarbonate ion	K⁺	potassium ion
Hct	hematocrit	KCL	potassium chloride
HCTZ	hydrochlorothiazide	kg	kilogram (1,000 grams; 2.2 pounds)
HEENT	head, eyes, ears, nose, and throat	KVO	keep vein open (30–60 µgtt/min)
HF	heart failure	L	left, liter
Hg	mercury	lb	pound
HIV	human immuno-deficiency virus	LLQ	left lower quadrant
HPI	history of present illness	LMP	last menstrual period
HR	heart rate	LOC	level of consciousness
hr., h	hour	LP	lumbar puncture
HTN	hypertension	LPM	liters per minute
Hx	history	LS	lung sounds
I&O	intake and output	LVAD	left ventricular assist device
ICD	implantable cardioverter defibrillator	LUQ	left upper quadrant
ICF	intracellular fluid	LZ	landing zone
ICP	intracranial pressure	m	meter
IDDM	insulin-dependent diabetes mellitus	MAOI	monoamine oxidase inhibitor
IL	intralingual	mcg	microgram (1/1,000,000 of 1 gram)
IM	intramuscular	MDI	metered dose inhaler
IO	intraosseous	mEq	milliequivalent
IPPB	intermittent positive pressure breathing	mg	milligram (1/1,000 of 1 gram)
*IU	*write out* international unit	Mg⁺⁺	magnesium ion
IUD	intrauterine device	*MgSO₄	*write out* magnesium sulfate
IV	intravenous	MI	myocardial infarction
IVP	intravenous push; intravenous pyelogram	Min/min	minute(s)
IVR	idioventricular rhythm	ml, mL	milliliter (1/1,000 of 1 liter; 1 mL)
JVD	jugular venous distension	mm	millimeter

* Unapproved abbreviation

MOI	mechanism of injury	PAC	premature atrial contraction
*MS, MSO₄	*write out* morphine sulfate	PAH	pulmonary arterial hypertension
MVA	motor vehicle accident	PASG	pneumatic antishock garment
N/V	nausea and vomiting	PAT	paroxysmal atrial tachycardia
NA	not applicable	p.c., pc	after meals
Na⁺	sodium ion	PCP	pneumocystis carinii
NaCl	sodium chloride	PCO₂	carbon dioxide pressure
NAD	no acute distress, no apparent distress	PE	physical exam
NaHCO₃	sodium bicarbonate	PEA	pulseless electrical activity
NB	newborn	PEARL	pupils equal and react to light
NG	nasogastric	PEEP	positive end-expiratory pressure
NIDDM	non-insulin-dependent diabetes mellitus	PETCO₂	partial pressure of end-tidal carbon dioxide
NKA	no known allergy	pH	hydrogen ion concentration (inverse)
NPO	nothing by mouth	PICC	peripherally inserted central catheter
NRB	non-rebreather (mask)	PID	pelvic inflammatory disease
NS	normal saline (0.9%)	PLA	Plasma-Lyte-A
NSAID	non-steroidal anti-inflammatory drug	PMH	past medical history
NSR	normal sinus rhythm	PND	paroxysmal nocturnal dyspnea
NTG	nitroglycerin	P.O., p.o., po	by mouth, orally
O₂	oxygen	PO₂	oxygen pressure
OB	obstetrics	POC	position of comfort
OD	overdose	POCT	point-of-care testing
OLMC	online medical control	PP	postpartum
oz	ounce	PPM	permanent pacemaker
p̄	after	PR, pr	per rectum; rectally

* Unapproved abbreviation

PRN, prn	as needed	S$_a$O$_2$	arterial oxygen saturation
PSM	pulse, sensory and motor functions	SAH	subarachnoid hemorrhage
PSVT	paroxysmal supra-ventricular tachycardia	SBP	systolic blood presure
Pt., pt	patient	SC, SQ	subcutaneous
PVC	premature ventricular contraction	SL	sublingual
q	every	SLUDGE	salivation, lacrimation, urination, defecation, gastrointestinal distress, emesis
*Q.D., QD	*write out* every day	SOB	short of breath
qh	every hour	SpO$_2$	saturation via pulse oximetry
qid	four times a day	SQ	subcutaneous
*Q.O.D., QOD	*write out* every other day	S/S, S/Sx	signs and symptoms
R	right	stat	immediately
RBC	red blood cell	STD	sexually transmitted disease
RL	Ringer's lactate solution	Sx	symptoms
RLQ	right lower quadrant	Sz	seizure
R/O or RO	rule out	T	temperature
ROM	range of motion	TB	tuberculosis
RR	respiratory rate	TCA	tricyclic antidepressant
RSI	rapid-sequence intubation	TIA	transient ischemic attack
RUL	right upper lobe	tid	three times a day
RUQ	right upper quadrant	TKO	to keep open (30–50 µgtt/min)
Rx	prescription, therapy, treatment	Torr	millimeters of mercury (mm Hg)
s̄	without	TPR	temperature, pulse, and respiration
S-A, SA	sinoatrial	TQ	tourniquet

* Unapproved abbreviation

* Unapproved abbreviation

TX	therapy	WNL	within normal limits
℞*	*write out* unit	WPW	Wolff-Parkinson-White (syndrome)
UA	urinalysis	wt	weight
URI	upper respiratory infection	×	times
UTI	urinary tract infection	yo, y/o, y.o.	years old
UV	umbilical vein	↓	decrease(d)
VAD	ventricular assist device	↑	increase(d)
V-Fib, VF	ventricular fibrillation	♂	male
VNS	vagus nerve stimulator	♀	female
VS	vital signs	µ	micro (1/1,000,000)
VT	ventricular tachycardia	∇	change (delta)
V-Tach	ventricular tachycardia	∅	no, none, null
VTE	venous thromboembolism	>	less than
/w	with	≤	less than or equal to
w/o	without	<	greater than
WBC	white blood cell	≥	greater than or equal to

■ Spell Checker

abdomen
abrasion
abruptio
  placenta
abscess
abuse
acetone
acidosis
accumulate
addiction
adolescent
afebrile
agonal
alcohol
alcoholic
alcoholism
alkali
alkalosis
aligned
alignment
allergy
alleviate
alopecia
Alzheimer
amenorrhea
aminophylline
ammonia
amnesia
amniotic
amphetamines
amputation
analgesic
anaphylactic

anaphylaxis
anemia
anemic
anesthesia
anesthetic
aneurysm
angulation
anorexia
antecubital
antibiotic
anticoagulant
antidepressant
antidote
antipyretic
antispasmodic
anxiety
anxious
aphasia
aphasic
antacid
antecubital
apnea
apneic
appearance
appendicitis
appendectomy
appendix
apprehensive
aqueous
arachnoid
arrhythmia
arteriosclerosis
arthritis
artifact
artificial

ascites
ashen
asphyxia
aspirate
aspiration
assault
assessment
asthma
asthmatic
asystole
atelectasis
atrial
aura
auscultate
auscultation
avulsion
axilla
axillary

B

babies
Babinski
bacteremia
bacterial
balance
bandage
barbiturate
barium
barotrauma
baseline
basal
basilar
basic
belch
belching

benign
Betadine
biceps
bicuspid
bifocal
bifurcate
bifurcation
bigeminal
bigeminy
bilateral
bile
biopsy
blackout
bladder
blindness
bolus
botulism
bowel
brachial
bradycardia
bradypnea
brain
breast
breath
breathe
breech
bronchi
bronchial
bronchiectasis
bronchiolitis
bronchitis
bronchospasm
bronchus
bruise
bruit

buccal
bulimia
bunion
bursitis
buttock

C

calcium
cancer
cannula
capillaries
capillary
carbon
carbon monoxide
cardiogenic
cardiopulmonary
cardiovascular
cardioversion
carotid
carpal
carpopedal
cartilage
casualty
cataract
catheter
caudal
cellulitis
cerebellum
cerebral
cerebral palsy
cerebrospinal
cerebrovascular
cerebrum
cervical
cervix
cesarean
characteristic
chemotherapy
Cheyne-Stokes
cholecystitis
cholesterol
circulation

cirrhosis
clavicle
coagulate
coccyx
colitis
collapse
Colles
colostomy
comatose
comminuted
communicable
concussion
congenital
congestion
congestive
conjunctiva
conjunctivitis
conscious
consciousness
constipation
constrict
constricted
contagious
contaminate
contraction
contraindication
contusion
convalescent
convulsion
copious
cornea
corneal
coronary
cranium
cranial
crepitus
cricoid
cricothyroid
cricothyrotomy
croup
cutaneous
cyanosis
cyanotic

cystic fibrosis
cystitis

D

deceleration
decerebrate
decompensate
decompression
decorticate
decubitus
defecate
defibrillate
defibrillation
deficiency
deficit
definitive
deformity
dehydrated
dehydration
delirious
delirium tremens
dementia
dependent
depression
dermatitis
development
dextrose
diabetes
diabetic
diagnosis
diaphoresis
diaphragm
diaphragmatic
diarrhea
diastolic
difficulty
digestion
digitalis
dilate
dilation
diminished
diplopia

discoloration
discomfort
disease
disentanglement
dislocated
dislocation
dispersed
disruption
dissecting
dissociation
dissolve
distal
distended
distention
diuretic
diverticulitis
dizziness
dorsalis pedis
duodenum
duration
dysarthria
dysconjugate
dysfunction
dysmenorrhea
dysphagia
dyspnea
dyspneic
dysrhythmia
dysuria

E

ecchymosis
eclampsia
ectopic foci
ectopy
edematous
electrolytes
emaciated
emboli
embolism
embolus
emesis
emetic

emphysema	failure	genital	herpes
emphysemic	faint	genitalia	hiccough
encephalitis	fallopian	genitals	hormones
endocarditis	Fahrenheit	geriatric	humerus
endotracheal	febrile	gestation	hyperextension
enteritis	fecal	gestational	hyperglycemia
enzyme	femoral	girdle	hyperkalemia
epidermis	femur	glaucoma	hyperpnea
epidural	fetal	glottis	hyperpyrexia
epiglottis	fetus	glucose	hyperreflexia
epiglottitis	fever	gonorrhea	hyperresonance
epilepsy	feverish	gout	hypertension
epileptic	fibrillate	grand mal	hyperventilation
epinephrine	fibrillation	grandeur	hyphema
epiphyseal plate	fibula	gravida	hypnotic
epistaxis	flaccid	groin	hypoglycemia
equilibrium	flail	gurney	hyporesonance
equivalent	flare		hypotension
esophageal	flaring	**H**	hypothermia
esophagus	flexed		hypoxia
etiology	flexible	hallucinate	hypoxic
eustachian	fontanelle	hallucination	hypovolemia
eviscerate	foramen	hallucinogen	hysterectomy
evisceration	magnum	hazard	hysteria
exacerbated	forearm	hazardous	
examination	forehead	Heimlich	**I**
excessive	fossa	hematemesis	
exhale	fracture	hematoma	idiosyncrasy
exhaust	frostbite	hematuria	idioventricular
exhaustion		hemiparalysis	ileum
expiration	**G**	hemiplegia	iliac crest
exposure		hemophilia	ilium
exsanguinate	gag reflex	hemopneumo-	immobilize
exsanguinating	gait	thorax	immobilization
external	gallbladder	hemoptysis	immunization
extremity	gallstone	hemorrhage	impairment
extricate	gangrene	hemorrhagic	impending
extrication	gastric	hemorrhoid	inadequate
extrude	gastritis	hemothorax	incident
eyeball	gastroenteritis	hepatitis	incision
	gastrointestinal	hepatomegaly	incontinence
F	gauge	hereditary	incontinent
	gauze	hernia	increment
facial	generalized	heroin	induced

indwelling
inebriated
inebriation
infarct
infarction
infection
infectious
inferior
infiltrate
infiltration
inflammation
infusion
ingestion
inguinal
inhalation
initiate
injection
inoculation
insensible
insufficiency
insufficient
insulin
integumentary
intercostal
intermittent
intestinal
intestine
intoxicated
intracranial
intracranial pressure
intramuscular
intravenous
intubate
intubation
ipecac
irreversible
irritability
ischemia
ischemic
ischial
ischium

J

jaundice
jejunum
joules
jugular
junctional
juvenile

K

keratitis
ketoacidosis
kidneys
kidney stones
knuckle
Kussmaul
kyphosis

L

laceration
laryngeal
laryngectomy
laryngoscope
laryngospasm
laryngitis
laryngospasm
larynx
lateral
lavage
lethargic
lethargy
leukemia
leukocytes
ligament
linear
lividity
localize
lumbar
lymph

M

malaise
malignant

malleolus
malnourished
mandible
maneuver
manifestation
marijuana
maxilla
measles
medial
meninges
meningitis
menstruation
mesenteric
mesentery
metabolism
metacarpal
midclavicular
minimal
minimum
mitral
Mobitz
modality
moderate
morbidity
morphine
mucosal
mucus
mucous
membrane
multifocal
multigravida
myalgia
myasthenia gravis
mydriasis
myocardial
myocardium

N

naloxone
narcosis
narcotic
nares

narrowing
nasogastric
nasopharyngeal
nausea
nauseated
nauseous
nebulizer
necrosis
necrotic
neonatal
neonate
neurogenic
neurologic
nitroglycerin
nocturia
nocturnal
noxious
nystagmus

O

obese
obesity
oblique
obstruct
obturator
occipital
occiput
occlude
occlusion
occlusive
ocular
odontoid
oliguria
opaque
ophthalmic
opiate
opposite
orbit
orbital
organophosphate
oriented
orifices
oropharyngeal

oropharynx
orthopedic
orthopnea
orthostatic
oscilloscope
osteoporosis
otitis
ovarian
ovaries
oxygenate
oxygenated

P

pacemaker
palate
pallor
palpate
palpation
palpitation
palsy
pancreas
pancreatitis
paradoxical
paralysis
paranoia
paranoid
paraplegia
paraplegic
parasympathetic
parenteral
paresthesia
parietal
paroxysmal
partial seizure
patella
patent
pathologic
patience
pectoris
pedal edema
pediatric
pelvic
penetrate

penicillin
peptic
percussion
perfuse
perfusion
pericardial
perineal
perineum
peripheral
peritoneum
peritonitis
personnel
perspiration
pertinent
petit mal
pharmacology
pharyngeal
pharynx
phenobarbital
phlebitis
phlegm
phobia
physiologic
pinna
placenta
previa
platelets
pleural
pneumonia
pneumothorax
poison
poisoning
polydipsia
polyphagia
polyuria
pontine
popliteal
posterior
postictal
postpartum
posture
potassium
potential

precordial
preeclampsia
pregnancy
pregnant
premature
prenatal
prescribe
presenting
previous
priapism
primigravida
primipara
prodromal
profuse
prognosis
prolapse
prone
prophylactic
prostate
prostatitis
prosthesis
proximal
pruritus
psychiatric
psychogenic
psychologic
psychosis
psychosomatic
puberty
pubis
pulmonary
pulsating
pulsation
pulseless
pulsus
pulsus alternans
puncture
pupillary

Q

quadrant
quadriplegia
quality

quivering

R

raccoon eyes
radial
radial pulse
radiates
radius
rales
rational
reaction
rebound
rectal
rectum
recumbent
recurrence
reduce
redness
reflex
refractory
regurgitate
regurgitation
rehydrate
relapse
relief
relieve
remission
renal
renal colic
resistance
respiration
respiratory
respond
response
restless
resuscitate
resuscitation
retention
retina
retraction
retrograde
retroperitoneal
retrosternal

rheumatic
rhonchi
rhythm
rhythmic
rigor
rigor mortis
rotate
rotating
route
routine
rubella
rupture

S

sacroiliac
sacrum
sagittal
salicylate
saliva
scapula
scar
sciatic
sclera
sebaceous
secondary
secrete
secretion
sedate
sedation
seize
seizure
Sellick
  maneuver
semi-Fowler
senile
sensation
sensitive
sensory
separation
sepsis
septic
septum

sequelae
sever
severe
severity
shallow
shiver
shortness
shoulder
sibling
sinus
skeletal
skull
sleepiness
sleepy
snoring
spasm
spastic
sphincter
spinous
spleen
splenomegaly
spontaneous
sprain
sputum
stability
stable
status
  asthmaticus
status
  epilepticus
stenosis
sterile
sternum
stethoscope
stimulate
stimuli
stimulus
stomach
straight
strain
stretch
stretcher

stridor
stroke
subclavian
subcutaneous
subdural
sublingual
substernal
successive
sudden
sufficient
suffocate
suicidal
suicide
superficial
supine
suppository
supraventricular
swallow
sweat
swelling
swollen
symmetric
symmetrical
symmetry
sympathetic
symphysis pubis
symptom
symptomatic
syncopal
syncope
syndrome
syphilis
syringe
syrup
systemic
systolic

T

tachycardia
tachypnea
tamponade
tarsals

technique
teeth
telemetry
temperature
temporal
temporo-
  mandibular
tenderness
tendon
tension
tetanus
tetany
toxoid
therapeutic
thoracic
thorax
thready
throat
thrombi
thrombosis
thrombus
thumb
thyroid
tibia
tibial
tuberosity
tincture
tingling
tinnitus
tissue
titrate
tolerance
tolerate
tongue
tonic
tonsil
tonsillectomy
tonsillitis
tooth
tourniquet
toxemia
toxic

trachea
tracheostomy
traction
tranquilizer
transfusion
transient
transverse
trauma
tremors
Trendelenburg
triage
triangular
tricyclic
trigeminy
trousers
tuberculosis
tympanic

U

ulcer
ulceration
ulna
umbilical
umbilicus
unconscious
unifocal
unsynchronized

uremia
ureters
urethra
urethral
urinary
urinate
urine
urticaria
uterine
uterus
uvula

V

vaccine
vagal
vagina
vaginal
vallecula
Valsalva
varices
vas deferens
vascular
vasodilate
vasodilation
vasodilator
vasopressor
vasovagal

vehicle
vein
venereal
venipuncture
venous
ventilate
ventilation
ventilator
ventilatory
ventricle
ventricular
Venturi mask
vertebra
vertebrae
vertigo
vessels
viable
victim
viral
virus
viscera
visceral
vision
vitamins
volume
vomit
vomiting

vomitus
vulva

W

waist
weak
weakness
weight
wheal
wheeze
wheezing
widening
withdrawal
worsen
worsening
wrist

X

xiphoid

Y

yawn
yeast

Z

zygoma
zygomatic arch

■ Phone Numbers

911 Communication Center	
American Red Cross	
Chemtrec Emergency	1-800-424-9300
Chemtrec Nonemergency	1-800-262-8200
Child Protective Services	
Crisis Center	
Domestic Violence Shelter	
Employee Assistance Program	
HazMat Team	
Homeless Shelter	
Medical Examiner/Coroner	
Medical Resource Center	
National Response Center	1-800-424-8802
Organ Donation Center	
Poison Control Center	1-800-222-1222
Public Health Department	
Sexual Abuse Hotline	
State/County EMS Office	
Suicide and Crisis Lifeline	988
Translation Services	
Trauma Center	
Other	
Other	
Other	
Other	
Other	

Spanish Translations

(In Spanish, "h" is silent; "ll" is pronounced like "y" [yip]; "j" like "h" [ham]; "qu" like "k" [keep]; and "ñ" like "nya" [canyon]. An accented vowel [á, ó, etc.] simply indicates the syllable that must be stressed when pronouncing the word.)

History and Examination	
I am a paramedic (fire fighter, nurse, doctor).	Soy paramédico/paramédica (bombero/bombera, enfermera/enfermero, médico/médica).
I speak a little Spanish.	Hablo un poco de español.
Is there someone here who speaks English?	¿Alguien habla inglés?
What is your name?	¿Cómo se llama usted?
I don't understand.	No entiendo.
Can you speak more slowly please?	¿Puede hablar más despacio, por favor?
Wake up sir/madam.	Despiértese, señor/señora.
Sit up.	Siéntese.
Listen.	Escúcheme.
How are you?	¿Cómo se siente?
Do you have neck or back pain?	¿Le duele el cuello o la espalda?
Were you unconscious?	¿Estuvo inconsciente?
Move your fingers and toes.	Mueva los dedos de las manos y los pies.
What day is today?	¿Qué día es hoy?
Where is this?	¿Dónde estamos?

Where are you?	¿Dónde está usted?
What is your telephone number? … address?	¿Cuál es su número de teléfono? … domicilio?
When were you born?	¿Cuándo nació?
Sit here please.	Siéntese aquí, por favor.
Lie down please.	Acuéstese, por favor.
Do you have pain? … trouble breathing? … weakness?	¿Tiene dolor? … dificultad para respirar? … debilidad?
Where?	¿Dónde?
Show me where it hurts with your hand.	Muéstreme con su mano dónde le duele.
Does the pain increase when you breathe?	¿El dolor aumenta al respirar?
Breathe deeply through your mouth. Breathe slowly …	Respire profundo por la boca. Respire lentamente …
What medicine(s) do you take?	¿Qué medicina(s) toma?
Have you been drinking?	¿Ha estado tomando alcohol?
Have you taken any drugs?	¿Ha tomado alguna droga?
Do you have chest pain? … heart problems? … diabetes? … asthma? … allergies?	¿Tiene dolor en el pecho? … problemas del corazón? … diabetes? … asma? … alergias?
Have you had this pain before?	¿Ha tenido el mismo dolor en otras ocasiones?
How long ago?	¿Hace cúanto tiempo?
Are you sick to your stomach?	¿Tiene náuseas o asco?
Are you pregnant?	¿Está embarazada?

Do you need to vomit?	¿Quiere vomitar?
You will be okay.	Va a estar bien.
Everything will be okay.	Todo saldrá bien.
It is not serious.	No es grave.
It is serious.	Es grave.

Treatment	
Please don't move.	Por favor, no se mueva.
What's the matter?	¿Qué pasa?
Do you want to go to the hospital?	¿Quiere ir al hospital?
To which hospital?	¿A cuál hospital?
You must go to the hospital.	Tiene que ir al hospital.
We're going to take you to the hospital.	Le vamos a llevar al hospital.
We are going to give you oxygen.	Le vamos a poner oxígeno.
We are going to apply a C-collar.	Vamos a ponerle un collarín.
We are going to give you an IV.	Vamos a ponerle un suero.

Miscellaneous			
Thank you.	Gracias.	hand	la mano
Excuse me.	Disculpe.	head	la cabeza
Hello.	Hola.	heart	el corazón
Goodbye.	Adiós.	to help	ayudar
Yes.	Sí.	hip	la cadera
No.	No.	hypertension	hipertensión/ presión alta
abdomen	el abdomen	leg	la pierna
ankle	el tobillo	lungs	los pulmones
arm	el brazo	meds	las medicinas
back	la espalda	mouth	la boca

162

bone	el hueso	neck	el cuello
cancer	cáncer	penis	el pene
chest	el pecho	stretcher	la camilla
drugs	drogas	stroke	ataque cerebral
ear	el oído	throat	la garganta
eye	el ojo	vagina	la vagina
foot	el pie	wrist	la muñeca
fracture	una fractura		

■ Metric Conversions

Temperature	
°F	°C
106	41.1
105	40.6
104	40
103	39.4
102	38.9
101	38.3
100	37.8
99	37.2
98.6	37
98	36.7
97	36.1
96	35.6
95	35
94	34.4
93	33.9
92	33.3
91	32.8
90	32.2
89	31.7
88	31.1
87	30.6
86	30
85	29.4
84	28.9
83	28.3

Weight	
lbs	kg
396	180
374	170
352	160
330	150
308	140
286	130
264	120
242	110
220	100
209	95
198	90
187	85
176	80
165	75
154	70
143	65
132	60
121	55
110	50
99	45
88	40
77	35
66	30
55	25
44	20

Misc.

Length

39.4 in. = 1 m	
1 in. = 2.54 cm	
3/8 in. = 1 cm	

Weight

2.2 lb = 1 kg	
1 lb = 454 g	
1 oz = 28 g	
1 mg = 1,000 μg	
1 g = 1,000 mg	

"3:00 am Rule" for converting pounds to kilograms:
Divide pounds (lbs) by 2 and subtract 10%.

Volume

1 tsp = 5 mL	
1 tbsp = 15 mL	
1 fl oz = 30 mL	
1 qt = 946 mL	

Pressure

1 mm Hg = 1.36 cm H$_2$O	

Temperature

°F	°C
82	27.8
81	27.2
80	26.7
75	23.8
70	21.1
59	18.3
32	0

Weight

lbs	kg
33	15
22	10
15	7
11	5
7.5	3.5
5	2.3
3	1.4

CONTENTS

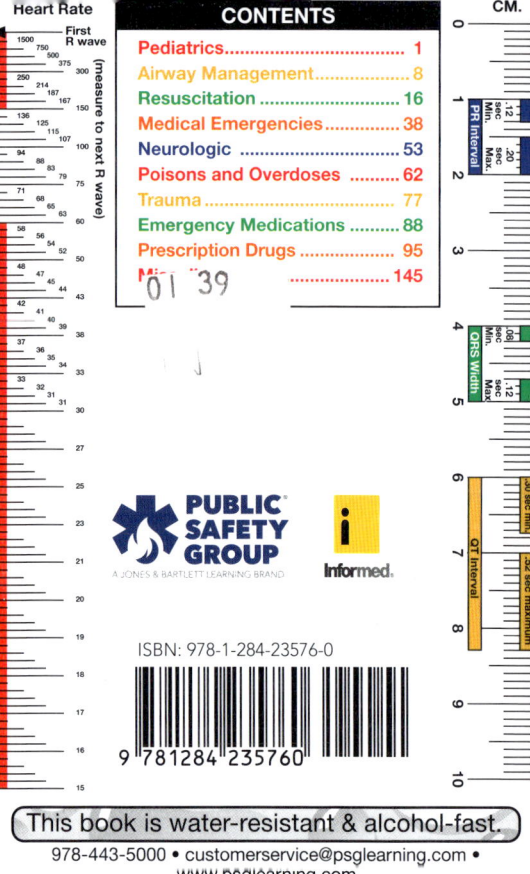

PR Interval .12 sec Min. .20 sec Max.

QRS Width .08 sec Min. .12 sec Max.

QT Interval :30 sec min | :50 sec maximum

PUBLIC SAFETY GROUP
A JONES & BARTLETT LEARNING BRAND

i Informed.

ISBN: 978-1-284-23576-0

9 781284 235760

This book is water-resistant & alcohol-fast.

978-443-5000 • customerservice@psglearning.com •
www.psglearning.com